Living Naturally

Viv Turner

Three Trees Press
Dudley
West Midlands

© Viv Turner 1993

Published in Great Britain in 1993 by

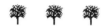

Three Trees Press
Dudley
West Midlands

Cover illustration by Tony Ball
Printed and bound in Great Britain

ISBN 0–9521144–0–2

Note from the Publisher
Any information given in this book is not intended to be taken as a
replacement for medical advice. Any person with a condition
requiring medical attention should consult a qualified medical
practitioner or suitable therapist.

Contents

Page

Dedication   i
Acknowledgments   ii
Foreword by Norman Gifford M.B.E.   iii
Chief coach at Sussex County Cricket club.
Former Captain of Worcestershire and Warwickshire
County Cricket Clubs and test match cricketer.

Chapter

1	Awareness of Ill Health	1
2	Animal Rights	11
3	All Alone	17
4	Homoeopathy	21
5	Helen	26
6	The Bristol Diet	29
7	Will to Live	37
8	Search for Dlet	43
9	Food Combining	56
10	My Lifetime Diet	60
11	Exercise and Fresh Air	86
12	Nature	94
13	Faith	105
14	Mind Elevation	111
15	Stress	123
16	Natural First Aid	133
17	People	151
18	Wolff-Parkinson-White Syndrome	163
19	Lesley	182

20	Natural Healing	187
	Spiritual Healing	187
	Relaxation	189
	Reflexology	194
	Chromotherapy	197
	Crystal Therapy	207
	Hypnosis	221
	Massage	226
	Hydrotherapy	232
	Metamorphosis	239
	Reiki	243
21	Grief	251
22	Self Love	255
	Epilogue	259

For Dai

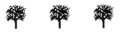

ACKNOWLEDGMENTS

I should like to express my thanks to Brian for patiently checking my original manuscript and to Bernice, who shared my early school years, for typing my often illegible notes with much patience. Without Brian and Bernice, my story would never have been told.

I acknowledge the artistic talents of Tony Ball in creating my cover illustration.

I am indebted to Hasnain Walji for his assistance in publishing my story for which I shall always be grateful.

I wish to thank Ned Williams for his guidance and support.

FOREWORD

Viv and I have been friends for many years and she has always been interested in my physical fitness and that I maintained this with a sensible lifestyle including wholesome food, fresh air and of course plenty of exercise. She often commented on the fact that I never suffered from coughs and colds and had an abundance of energy.

On reading her story I am pleased that in many ways she has followed my guidelines and I am sure that this book will assist many people who wish to become healthy using natural methods.

I wish her good luck and health and happiness in the future.

Norman Gifford M.B.E.

1

AWARENESS OF ILL HEALTH

Cancer came into my life during the hot summer of 1984. On many occasions I had considered this most dreaded possibility but always managed to shut my mind to it, ignoring nagging pains that never quite disappeared before pushing to the fore again and the awful feeling of unwellness and lassitude that was now a daily occurrence.

In August 1984 I was on holiday with my family in Criccieth North Wales, where we had spent annual holidays for many years. Three precious weeks to be looked forward to throughout the year and up until then every minute savoured with enjoyment. The superb view from the gentle ruins of Criccieth's Castle over the wide sweep of Tremadog Bay to mighty Harlech Castle towering in grandeur and ending in the flat distance of Mochras Island could not now dull the gnawing pain. As I sat on the lawn of the house that we had hired, listening to the lap of the waves only yards away feeling the warmth of the sun on my skin, I knew that I could not ignore my waning health any longer.

Summer is always a busy time with my young son Jamie on school holiday. Yet, my recurring gynaecological disorders that I kept pushing from my mind in the wish that they would recede permanently, always returned with renewed vigour until my only awareness was of dull pain and a bodily feeling of great coldness. All of my life I had never been plagued with the so called feminine problems. My body always working like clockwork, this condition was new to me. I put it down to stress, overwork, being unable to relax, and tried to convince myself that this holiday was all that was needed to put me right.

1

We retraced our steps over familiar ground. The wonderful walk was along the wide shingle beach to Black Rock with the calm shimmering sea on one side and the rolling green hills dotted with sheep on the other, only this time I could not complete the walk. We made our annual visit to Llanystumdwy Farm where we could feed the animals and have a ride in the farm cart and gaze to the distant sea. I listened to the Welsh singing that was always heard at the farm and as I held a timid rabbit close to me I derived no comfort from its warmth as all that I was aware of was how ill I felt. We walked along the banks of the Afon Dwyfor, following in the footsteps of that great statesman David Lloyd George and when I looked up to where his body lay in the place where he had chosen to be buried, for the first time I felt the cold chill of death.

Our holiday over, we returned home and the beginning of September saw the start of a new school year. Jamie had his school life and friends to absorb him and my husband Brian a busy office. I had time to myself and my rapidly worsening health. Constant pain in my lower abdomen and a steady weight loss left me gaunt and haggard. People looked at me with concern and I could tell hesitated to ask how I was. By this time I was feeling too ill to do anything but endeavour to cope with increasing difficulty with a normal day.

In October I went to see my General Practitioner who gave me a cervical smear test and said the result would be in shortly and then I should make an appointment to see him. I waited the required time and was told that it had not returned but was reassured that everything must be fine or the result would be in by now. When it did arrive it was as I had feared abnormal and my doctor arranged for me to see a gynaecologist. This I did and had an examination and talk with the consultant who agreed that there was something wrong with me. He confirmed what my General Practitioner had said that I had an erosion of the womb which was inflamed and bled when touched and he strongly recommended that I enter hospital for further investigation under anaesthetic for more positive diagnosis. As far as he had been able to discover at this stage he said that my problem could have arisen due to instruments used during the epidural birth of Jamie. He felt it more likely to be a polyp which could be malignant and if it was and was left untreated, within six months I would be past all help. I had requested that he be entirely honest with me and he had done this. He continued to stress the seriousness of my condition and that I agree to him arranging for me to enter hospital. I respected the surgeons advice but declined to make a decision then and said that I would discuss it with my family and again visit my General Practitioner.

I returned home and made an appointment to see my General Practitioner again and that evening had a family discussion. The immediate reaction was to do as the gynaecologist had urged, he being a most respected local surgeon who had left me in no doubt of what my future could be.

The next day I saw my General Practitioner. I am most fortunate in having a doctor who will always give one as much time as one needs. There is no rushing in and out of patients, a light airy consulting room and large bright waiting area. There were three doctors in the practice. To this day one I have never seen and the second only on one occasion as I hardly ever visited my medical advisers under normal circumstances. My doctor listened to what I had to say and was concerned when I told him of my decision not to enter hospital where the minimum treatment that I would have would be a womb scrape and the bleeding areas cauterised. He was understanding and suggested that, at least, I have regular smear tests to keep a check on the irregularities. He also said that should I change my mind he would immediately make the necessary arrangements for me to enter hospital. I promised to do this and do feel most fortunate to have such a considerate doctor. I went out into the waiting area, looking apologetically at the patients as I had greatly overstayed the stipulated five minutes. I said goodbye to the receptionists, the pleasantest of girls always smiling and helpful.

I came home. Now that the decision had been made and accepted I felt that I could look forward in my chosen way, rather than do as orthodox medicine dictated.

In 1981 at just sixty six years of age my Mother had died after a two and a half year fight with cancer. Her death certificate stated 'Metastatic carcinoma rectum' which explains a great deal but not the agony and indignities that she bore with such fortitude. In December 1978 she had a bowel irregularity that did not give her pain but that she mentioned to her General Practitioner who recommended that she see a local surgeon. This she did and was told that she had a small polyp in her rectum that was benign and that a small operation would sort the problem out for her. Being reassured she agreed to enter hospital before Christmas to get it 'all over' and the day of her operation soon arrived. The pre-operation bowel wash-outs seemed severe to me for a minor operation but we were assured that it was all normal practice. I telephoned the hospital to be told that she had had the operation and could be visited. My father was the first person to see her and at her request suggested that I wait until she was a little better before I visited her. This did not greatly alarm me as my mother always thought of others before herself and I thought was probably still drowsy from the anaesthetic. Nothing could have prepared me for how I found her as in no way did I delay my visit to her. On the way along the corridor to the ward I passed some of the nurses who looked rather uncomfortable when they saw me. So many of them I knew well from the years I had worked in that hospital. In the long ward my mother's bed was adjacent to the sister's office. I knelt beside her in horror and fear of what I was seeing. She looked so ill but in a whisper told me not to worry and she would be fine and home as soon as possible. The words that I spoke I don't recall, only her constant reassurance that the doctors would make her better and not to worry. From entering the hospital looking well she now looked haggard and drawn and after visiting hour I sought out the duty nurse who would tell me nothing but referred me to the sister who likewise told me nothing and referred me to the doctor. He was not available and the start of a nightmare two and a half years had begun.

Eventually my mother came home after many weeks in hospital. Her minor operation had been a colostomy that I had never heard of. I was reassured by the medical personnel involved that the polyp that had been removed was non-malignant and that the colostomy had only been necessary due to its situation in the bowel.

For the rest of my mother's life she was never able to sit without constant pain but still she had faith in her medical advisers. Life consisted of daily visits from the district nurse who was a great source of strength to us all. From being an attractive lady she gradually became attenuated and as time went on the pain increased.

During the summer of 1979 we persuaded her to come on holiday to Criccieth with us. She was undecided as she did not want to be a burden to us, but somehow we managed it, using two cars and all the items that were necessary to look after a stoma. It was a holiday tinged with sadness as she was only able to take a short daily walk of a few yards beyond our holiday home. She didn't see the beauty of the hills or feel the warmth of the sun as her life was becoming too painful to notice anything other than her failing health. We returned home after what was to be her last holiday and she did less and less, until my father took over all household work with as much help from me as was possible. She became so tired and ill we had to ask her doctor for help.

He came to see her and said that she must see the surgeon again when we were told that another operation was needed immediately. As my mother suffered from angina it was felt that it was not advisable for her to have a general anaesthetic and that the operation would be performed during an epidural local spinal injection. My mother told me afterwards how her eyes were bandaged and how she could hear the surgeon talking to his assistants while she bravely endured this further ordeal.

She came home and in spite of the comforting words from all the medical people involved nothing could now hide my mother's piteous condition. As soon as she was able she saw her surgeon who told her that she needed radium followed by chemotherapy. At this point he had assumed that she knew that she had cancer. Neither she nor us had ever been told. None of us had come into close contact with the illness before. We knew nothing about radium or chemotherapy. I decided it was time I learned for myself so that I could do all in my power to help my mother. I first arranged to see my mother's surgeon without mentioning it to either of my parents. He was a charming gentleman whom I had learned to know well during my years in the health service. His secretary showed me into his quiet consulting room and I sat opposite him at his large desk and I said as an only child of a dear mother I wanted to know all that had happened. He told me that the polyp removed at her first operation necessitating the colostomy had been cancerous. He thought he had removed it all but obviously he could not have done so and the second operation had shown that this had spread. The second operation had been extensive and he could not be sure that he had removed all the cancerous cells and this was why he was suggesting radium and chemotherapy. I asked him what were my mother's survival chances and he said fifty-fifty. She had been told that this second operation had been for an abcess. I sadly took my leave of the surgeon. He was a kind and good man and I know that it could not have been easy for him to be so honest with me but I know that he had at all times done his best for my mother.

Thoughts went through my head as I drove home. What would have happened if she had had radium after her first operation, and if she had had chemotherapy. Why had we not been told the truth initially when we had asked? So many thoughts raced through my mind of no help now. I vowed that I would find out all that I could as no-one had a greater fighting spirit than my mother, so I went to the local library and took out all the books that I could find on cancer and its treatment. I read of the dreadful burning caused by radium but that it could be locally effective. I read of the dreadful sickness and hair loss caused by chemotherapy that could help in metastatic cancer. I read Dr. Joseph Issels book *Conquering Cancer* and of his great faith in chemotherapy and had wild ideas of taking my mother to his Clinic in France. I learned a great deal and still hid my awful secret of my mother's survival chances from my parents. I encouraged her to attend hospital for radium treatment, saying how fortunate we were to have a hospital so close. She coped with the required sessions of radium but it took a dreadful toll on her general health. The chemotherapy, when it came, was to change her life for ever. She said nothing tasted as it should and although she never lost her hair she became attenuated and lost her appetite. Most of her time was spent in bed. I sat with her many afternoons. My main desire was to encourage her to try to get better, but as I sat there as she lay quietly in bed I could see that she was losing all faith in her treatment and one afternoon as we sat together and looked through the window at the almond tree in the garden, brightly pink in the sun, she said she doubted she would see that tree flower again. I knew that she was trying to help me face up to the inevitable loss of the dearest of mothers and greatest of friends. Even then I could not accept that I would lose her.

Another hospital now became part of our lives and how could we know that the ward that we came to know so well during the ensuing months was associated with cancer and the dying. We were to meet a radiologist there who was to help her for the remainder of her life. He visited her at home on many occasions and we came to know each other quite well. Often my mother needed to enter hospital for blood transfusions after blood tests. The nurses on the ward were wonderful girls and a great help at that time to me. We came to know many patients. Most of them were not to go home but to die and after a blood transfusion and hospital hair shampoo I told myself how much better my mother looked than they did. My mother did all that she could to keep me cheerful, telling me that she was only sixty five and would get better. Many times she had told me that her mother had died when she was only thirty seven and how lucky I was that this would not happen to me. Of course I believed her. I wanted to more than anything. During the summer of 1980 when our annual family holiday was out of the question, I asked her during a stay in hospital whether she would like to spend a few weeks at my home which would be a change for her. This immediately gave her a mental lift as she had never stayed at my present home where we had only been a short time. Arranging for her stay was therapeutic for us all as it was something to look forward to and pleasurable to arrange. It would give my father a well earned rest from housekeeping which he had never had to do during his married life but which he coped with admirably. The house was re-arranged to make life easy for my mother. The most comfortable chair was placed in the sunniest part of the lounge. All her medical needs were arranged in her bedroom. Treasured photographs were brought for her dressing table. I was tense on the day that my father brought her home from hospital. I did so want everything to be just right. The car was brought as close to the front door as possible. With difficulty she walked into the house with our aid. Her happy smile masking the weariness of the journey, she thankfully rested in the chair covered in cushions to ease her pain. She looked so frail and thin. Long fingers were just bones and for many months she had worn no rings as they were all now too large and would fall off.

I did all that I could to make her stay a happy one, but the depth of her illness was apparent and could not be hidden when we were together all the time. By now she had no appetite and found all food tasted "horrible". She said it was all like poison and even a cup of tea was left hardly touched. On the sunny days she sat well wrapped in the garden and on her better days we walked as much as she could. Always a favourite pastime we both loved watching nature take its course but this summer was different. She did not comment on the bright blooms and for the first time did not plan the flowers that we should grow for the next year. Her stay with me had been a good one and had enabled her to see old friends as well as new faces and she said it was like coming home again back to the house where she had spent so much time as a young girl as the house had belonged to a close friend and her uncle and aunt had lived only a house away.

The holiday drew to a close and we did not talk of the next time. None of us could be so unkind and hypocritical of the truth but I am grateful for those hours we were to spend together as we had many a quiet talk that were to give me some comfort in the bleak times when she would never come again.

I always telephoned my father each morning and had a dreadful foreboding when one day he told me that my mother had been sick and she had only had cornflakes. This was so unlike my mother that I knew that this was a new phase of her illness and that I hoped it would not last as I knew that although she could endure unbelievable pain and was the bravest person she hated being sick. The sickness continued to the point where she carried a bowl when she visited hospital for her chemotherapy. She told me that she could not cope with it any more and by now found the treatment worse than the illness. The radiologist accepted her decision and agreed she was right to discontinue the chemotherapy. We always seemed to be travelling to or from that hospital and sitting waiting for visiting hour to start and trying to cheer my mother. She said that God was with her and she was not afraid. By now she had lost faith in all the medications but never her faith in God. She told me that she wanted so much to live. She had so much to live for and delighted in my young son Jamie.

At the end of 1980 I caught the mumps from Jamie who had recently started school. He had it mildly but I had it badly. I was unable to see my mother and not even able to speak on the telephone. My doctor said that there was no treatment so I just coped. Even to drink from a straw was painful until I started to improve and graduated to custard and porridge. For this Christmas my mother decided that I needed a change and insisted that we spend Christmas Day at her house as in no way could I have coped. With my father's help she gave us a wonderful meal that she did not enjoy and was hardly then able to eat, but to me it was the most significant meal and most well remembered for all the trouble she had taken as she wanted to thank me for all that I had done for her. We were all tearful and emotional but we had a happy time and were all very close. Brian often took her to hospital for check ups and she called him her son as she said a real one could not have been more of a help to her. It pleased me greatly to see this relationship and I will always be glad for them and ever appreciative of the part that Brian played in her darkest hours.

As is so often the case, the end comes unexpectedly. My mother had been told that she needed a blood transfusion. Just a few weeks before she had persuaded me to go away for a week's holiday as she was sufficiently stable for us to go. By now we were all feeling the strain and the thought of a week by the sea after two years would be such a relief. She said that she would miss us but was most insistent that we go.

She entered hospital and on that evening the 15the May 1981 my father received a telephone call to go at once. She died before he could reach the hospital. The shock waves engulfed me as I went with Brian to the hospital. On this so familiar route I kept thinking I was thirty seven years old.

So many thoughts crowded into my mind at that time founded on bewilderment and despair, but some memories always stayed to be clung to for comfort in my aloneness. Never during the past two and a half years had I ever not been given my mother's welcoming smile, for however she felt, her main concern was for her family. Sitting beside her on the side of the bed supporting her with one hand and holding the familiar bowl in the other, through her dressing gown one day her thin shoulders would shake and I would look in surprise to see her face brimming with laughter at the comic picture we must make. We were very close at this time and we would sit warm in the sun looking out onto the lawn where we would never sit together again and gossip girl talk as we had done all our lives. We daily watched the almond tree come into bud and the great joy to us when it opened into its soft delicate flower. That Spring I felt that the tree opened especially early just for her and gave her so much pleasure. The petals were more pink than ever before and the sun shone brighter through the bedroom window making the room warm and inviting and a place of haven and security. It was the room that I had had when I lived at home - for to me my parents house was always home - and I was glad that she was able to share its lightness and on good days look into the garden and be part of all the new life growing.

This time seemed divided with the hospital and we did joke about which bed she would have in the ward and of course it soon came to the time that she had been in them all. We made friends with other patients and the nurses and my mother forged friendships with a number of them. All were drawn together in a bond of uncertain life. So many times I counted the tiles on the floor as I waited in corridors impatiently to see her, nearly always in sunshine that I was grateful for as tears of rain I could not have tolerated. The eagerness of our meetings, when sitting close and sharing our days small news we politely but definitely shut out the other people in the ward, patients and visitors. This was our time and we did not accept anything encroaching on our togetherness. Time does dull the initial emotional gulf of shock and loss and the desperate hours recede and the happy times come to the fore. Lots of happy memories are always there to sustain the dark hours and the feel of my mother's hand and sound of her voice are real and always with me. Over the years the happy times helped me to cope and it was always with a sense of shock that I found I could laugh again, enjoy life and make plans for a future without my mother. Our perfect time together would live with me always and she had enriched my life and I realised that in so many ways I was fortunate.

We went down cold corridors to where she was lying alone. Her face looked contorted in pain and so aged and not like my precious mother. Later I was to see her just before her funeral, then so peaceful and serene. I sat for a while with Brian and held her cold and unresponsive hand. We went home and I arranged to see her consultant. It was a bright clear day with the sun shining and the cherry trees so bravely in bloom. So much had happened since she had told me a year ago that she would never see them again. I was welcomed into the consulting room by this kind and sympathetic man. He talked to me for a long time, quietly explaining that my mother had been beyond his help when he had met her and all that he had done for her had only been palliative. He said I must be glad for her that she had died so suddenly when her tired heart could not cope any more. For what she would have had to endure should she have lived, he knew I would not have wished for her. He said that he did not think that she could have had much longer to live and I took comfort in his words. He told me that the most precious gift that we have is our life and that I must go out and live. I had a father and husband and son who all needed me and I knew that I needed them. I had learned so much during the two and a half years of my mother's illness. It was a nightmare that I would have given my soul not to live through but it had taught me many things. I had to look after my own special life and let no-one but myself control it. I knew with certainty that the path that my mother had mistakenly and misguidedly taken with such trust and faith would never be for me. In making this decision I knew that she had not died in vain.

2

ANIMAL RIGHTS

October 13th 1982 was a momentous day for me for it was to open my eyes to a world that I knew little about and should be abolished for ever. It was the day of the first meeting of Dudley Animal Aid Group started by an enterprising and dedicated young couple, Tony and Phil. Over the ensuing years their total involvement to eradicate all animal suffering and to bring their pitiful plight to the notice of the general public left a lasting impression on me. I joined the group to help the animals and in doing so learned how to save myself.

A friend of mine, Angie in Criccieth, had first informed me of the existence of anti-vivisection societies when I had enquired about a car sticker that she had on her caravanette. I was immediately given copies of *Outrage*, the magazine of Animal Aid, many leaflets and posters. That summer holiday was marred by what I learned and during our time together we spent days parked on the promenade in the caravanette which was completely covered with posters and a stall to sell various items for the animal cause. This was my initiation into persuading other people to give some time and effort for helpless animals. At that time I read from the various leaflets to any interested parties but it was not long before I could recite the horrors without prompting. During that hot holiday the crowds did take an interest in us and like myself the majority were totally ignorant of the vivisectors evil trade. I felt that this was a cause that I could believe in and before returning home promised Angie that I would join an anti-vivisection group should I find one locally.

It was with much interest that October when I was introduced to Val, a cousin of my friend Chris. We had an immediate rapport. Both of us enjoyed travelling and were inquisitive of life

11

and she told me of the newly formed Dudley Animal Aid Group. She lived in Australia with her husband and as she was only here on a holiday that was drawing to a close I soon realised that I would not see much of her. The quality of our friendship overcame time and I joined her on the animal rights campaign.

Val was also a practising Buddhist about which I knew nothing. She explained this to me and gave me books to read. To her it meant a peaceful non-violent life to all living things and trying to be helpful to others. She was also a vegetarian and was horrified to learn that I ate meat and fish. It was against all her beliefs to kill even for food. Her father had been a butcher and as a child she had hated to see animal carcasses hung in his shop as she felt that the animals had as much right to live out their natural lives as humans. At this time it did not occur to me that eating animals was wrong and that was in no way connected with vivisection which like her I abhorred.

In the short time before she left for Australia we spent as much time as possible together, getting to know each other and realising how much we had in common as people as well as the bond of animal rights. I will always be grateful to her for introducing me to the Dudley Group and also for explaining Buddhism to me for I believe much of its teachings. She came into my life and helped give me something to believe in when I most needed it.

I read Hans Reusch book *Slaughter of the Innocent*, a penetrating account of the crime of this century, the evil life of the vivisector with total power over his victims. So many of these horrific deaths were supposedly in the cause of medical enlightenment. I read *Fettered Kingdoms* by John Bryant and many more books and wondered at mans sadistic role played out to always have the same unacceptable end. God did not put any of his creatures on this earth to be treated this way for any reason and I knew that no good would ever come from it. The Thalidomide, Opren and many more scandals confirm this.

My involvement with the group in its early stages was a happy one – leafletting in the town centre on chill winter days but enjoying the comradeship that comes in a group of people drawn together dedicated to a common cause. We held the usual fund raising jumble sales and had stalls at local fêtes. The group grew and we all began to question ourselves. I had a real fur coat that I wore with pleasure but the work of Fur Action Group made me stop and think of the animals that had died to give me something secondhand and bloodstained. I thought of foxes reared in this country in tiny cages in filthy conditions, their tethered existences solely to please woman's vanity and of animals trapped in the wild, forced to gnaw their own limbs in a bid for freedom but more likely to die caught with vicious metal teeth in their agonised bodies. Either way the end was the same. When I became aware of this suffering I never wore animal fur again.

Most of us became members of Animal Aid, British Union for the Abolition of Vivisection, Compassion in World Farming and many more organisations. Often we had speakers from these groups give talks about their work and how we could help and as we became more involved our interest grew in groups like the Hunt Saboteurs. On one humid never to be forgotten summer evening we crammed into the room booked for our meetings with great expectation for the guest speaker was to be Ronnie Lee, founder of the Animal Liberation Front. I had expected someone large and powerful and was rather disappointed to see this well known name a mild mannered young man in glasses and softly spoken. Our whispering stilled as he began to speak and the overhead claps of thunder and rain beating on the windows in no way drew our attention from him. He told us of the founding of the group known as The Band of Mercy but the name of which had been changed as it sounded like the Salvation Army. His humour was infectious and eased the tension in the packed hot room. His sincerity in dedicating his life to direct action was accepted by us all after his frustrating years of working for animals the legal way and his feeling of banging his head on a brick wall. To us all there was no crime in entering high security buildings to rescue animals. The only crime was that they were there at all. He was at great pains to inform us that the Animal Liberation Front was totally non-violent and no personal harm would come to anyone from them, not even the vivisectors themselves. After meeting Ronnie Lee it was ludicrous to imagine for a moment that he could harm anyone. That evening was a resounding success, for the Animal Liberation Front recruited many new members, including myself.

The Group's leaders worked incredibly hard to educate its members so that we could in turn teach others. This involved watching instructive films and one *Down on the Pig Farm* made a lasting impression on me. I learned of the tortured life of these intelligent animals forced to spend their entire existence on a concrete floor close bound with metal bars. Their tails were docked to stop "aggressive" behaviour which was pent up frustration when all the pigs wanted was freedom to move about as they were meant to do. We saw films showing calves taken from their mothers who cried pitifully. The poor animals were put into crates and kept confined and their miserable lives were cut short so that they could give humans the pleasure of white veal. Horses were transported abroad live and if they survived the journey they would be killed for human consumption. Sheep were crammed into large lorries to be taken to the slaughter house. The lot of the battery hen was so horrific its life belies belief. Animals leading unnatural lives and fed unnatural food were given injections which were supposedly necessary to keep them fit for human consumption.

The majority of the Group's members were vegetarians and some vegans and for the first time I questioned not only my right to eat animals but also whether this unwholesome food was doing me any good. My diet included all my personal delights, cream cakes, biscuits, all sweets and gallons of milk, bread plastered with butter and plenty of cheese. One member of the Group Trevor was determined to point out the error of my ways and explained how he had become a vegan and felt he was not only without guilt feelings that he had had when eating animal products but that his new diet was a more healthy one. He would always comment on the biscuits that I was constantly eating, asking did I read on the packet whether the ingredients were animal derived. I had to admit that I never gave it a thought and when he commented that the chocolate that I was never without was made with milk and didn't I realise that cows milk was for calves and not humans, particularly adult humans, I did pause and think. Why should I want food meant for a calf when in no way would I consider eating any kind of baby food.

My fellow members were encouraging when they knew that I wanted to alter my eating habits but found it laughable when I said that if I gave up all that they wanted me to I would soon starve as I had no idea what to put in its place and would they please tell me what I could eat. As expected the first item to be totally barred from consumption was meat of any kind followed closely by fish and in place of these I was to eat beans, lentils and nuts. Nuts I only ate at Christmas and the only beans that I ate were summer runner beans and what on earth were lentils and dried beans? This all seemed too much to cope with so I decided to settle for just eating as healthily as possible and joining the anti-vivisection societies would be my contribution for animal rights.

For some time I had frequented a new health shop intriguingly named *Foods of the Earth* that had recently been opened in my town by Dave and Moira a most enthusiastic couple who were eager to impart their knowledge and as they said – "help everyone to be healthy". Whenever I could I bought what had been organically grown and as these items had so much more flavour and were supposed to be better for me I was happy to change from my usual supermarket brands. I had for some time used a water filter for my tap water and found this made a great difference as I loved drinking water straight from the tap. I was encouraged in the health shop to try the bottled variety as I was told that this was more pure. I started with Malvern water that the Queen is reputed to drink and hated it. It seemed so heavy. I experimented and quickly realised how different waters can vary. The light French water was much to my liking and I drink only this water and do feel quite a connoisseur on the subject. Dave was a great help to me at this time with suggestions of items I should try. He was always interested in my comments. Over the months I tried many of the excitingly different foods he had to offer and he was always willing to order any items that I particularly wanted. I instinctively knew on trying Volvic mineral water that this suited me best and I had the satisfaction of recommending it to Dave. He agreed that it was a light drink and could appreciate my finding it so pleasingly palatable. In those early days I was deeply grateful for all the help I had from Dave and Moira. Like lots of people I had eaten white sliced bread for years and it took a lot of encouragement from Moira for me to try the granary bread that they had made up specially. I remember being given a mouthful in the shop and finding it so solid and hard to chew that it afforded them some amusement and me some embarrassment. I had no intention of consuming such a horrid concoction. To change the subject I said with some pride that I enjoyed cooking, particularly cakes and pies and was shown the brown wholewheat flour that I should use and brown unrefined sugar. I also purchased a variety of biscuits as these were eaten in large quantities in my home and felt that this was an encouraging start to my fitness campaign, but wondered was I really helping animals when I was told I could order from them free range chicken and also free range eggs. I was rather doubtful about this but although more expensive the eggs were delicious and the chicken of the most exquisite texture and delicate flavour and much appreciated by us all. We all found the biscuits rather chewy and if not as enjoyable as my usual brands they were palatable after a fashion.

My cakes seemed a most strange colour and no light texture as recommended by the experts, but smothered in icing and thickly filled with jam were edible, but I endured plenty of grumbles to stay as we were and what on earth had this to do with animals anyway.

My sponge puddings – usually so delicious with a thick coating of golden syrup were now rather like a heavy meal and only with a generous helping of custard were eaten and without enthusiasm.

Fruit pies were my most successful efforts with pastry rolled thinly but having a tendency to break and thickly filled with fruit. As we had a plentiful supply of rhubarb in the garden I spent days in the kitchen and soon had a well stocked freezer.

I made biscuits with wholemeal or stoneground flour but still used butter and with plenty of sugar these were quite popular.

My foray into the realms of healthy eating which included the doubtful eating of animals had only touched the tip of the iceberg when I gradually became aware of my increasing unwellness and in that Autumn of 1984 my life struggle was just beginning.

3

ALL ALONE

Mentally having decided to "go it alone" I was determined to succeed but physically I was deteriorating at an alarming rate. My weight was down to under 7 stones and at 5' 4" I was gaunt and haggard and from the concerned looks given me by anyone meeting me, particularly people who had not seen me recently, I knew that I was looking as ill as I felt. My appetite was poor and I was now sleeping badly. My energy seemed to be sapped daily and walking which had always been a constant source of pleasure was now a struggle which left me exhausted.

Brian started to take over the bulk of the shopping and he assisted my father in the daily trips to and from school with Jamie. I had help with my housework so had time to assess my pitiful condition. I went to see Phil the leader of our Animal Rights Group to inform her of my decision and say that I did not feel well enough to continue with the Group. She said that she admired my courage in refusing conventional medical advice and suggested two books that might help me – *The Bean Book* by Rose Elliot to help me become a vegetarian and *The Bristol Diet* by Dr. Alec Forbes which was now well known as a help to cancer patients. I also had a pile of Alternative Medicine and Diet books brought from the library.

Some I started and put down again. Some I read the odd chapter but being so listless and downhearted, I did begin to wonder: had I set myself such a mammoth task that I could not win? I was almost frightened to sleep in case I didn't wake up but I wanted to live and each morning I would lean on the window ledge and gaze at the park opposite my home and vowed that I would get better and that I would walk all round the park just as I did before I was ill.

Brian was busy at his office and was away long hours; Jamie was at school and enjoying his life and should in no way share my burden. My father had now renewed his acquaintance with old friends and found new ones and did not comprehend my situation. As I went out less and less I began to lose touch with many people that I had previously seen regularly. People whom I had considered friends didn't call. I was all alone. I went downstairs and lay on the settee.

At this critical point in my life my constant source of comfort was our family cat Mimi. She was a small golden brown tortoiseshell with pale green eyes and the most timid animal that I had ever known. All my life we had had a family cat and as an only child cats had been my friends as well as pets. All the cats had been so different and all much loved but Mimi was the kitten I had had when I moved into my own home. She was so quiet and frightened of strangers that most people thought her dull but to us she was to become the dearest sweetest natured cat in the world.

She was totally dependent on us for her wellbeing. She never caught mice or birds and her delight was to be in the warmth of our home and to be with us. She was most content to lie beside one of us and press her small body against ours. She never wanted to sit on laps – just to be close.

With the natural feline instinct she sensed that I needed her and before I was settled on the settee or on a chair or even on the days when I stayed in bed she would be with me. For hours she would give me the comfort of her presence and suffer me to cling to her and shed frightened tears onto her velvet fur. In those dark days her constant loving devotion was my sole consolation in my painful world.

She nestled against me as I lay on the settee and without enthusiasm picked up one book after another. All seemed to say eat natural foods as fresh as possible in as much variety as possible and plenty of seasonable vegetables and fruit. It was an effort to concentrate. The books were so positive – not an easy thing to be when every movement was an effort and it was so much easier to lie back and do nothing. So many hours we stayed together with my gaze on the woods at the rear of our garden, over the months seeing them change from bare cold wintry branches to the green leaves appearing with the coming of Spring when the birds sang and I felt I must make a start on my recovery.

Cooking was a great effort and the only meal that I did set as a goal was our traditional Sunday lunch that we shared with my father who always had a family Sunday with us since my mother had died. He enjoyed a roast joint and a good English lunch and as I did too I always managed to achieve this even though the price I paid in exhaustion afterwards was high. I did feel that we all needed this day together.

During the week the days were long and merged into the nights and I lost all count of time. I hardly walked at all as my legs felt so weak and I was covered in perspiration on any exertion.

My days started with hot strong tea with loads of sugar and toast thickly coated in butter and marmalade.

Mid-morning I would have strong coffee made with milk and again plenty of sugar and lunch times were usually something easy to prepare. I enjoyed cheese and crackers or cold meat sandwiches and now often had a dish of muesli with milk. Custard was still high on the list of enjoyable meals with quite a wide variety of choice from the freezer. I definitely enjoyed sweet items and thick jam sandwiches and a cream cake were popular and most evenings I enjoyed the delights of Mars bars and had a well stocked sweet tin containing most of the popular brands of chocolate.

I found cooked meals rather heavy even though I did one daily for Brian who always came in from the office wanting a proper dinner. I enjoyed jacket potatoes sometimes covered in butter with plenty of salt and sometimes with sliced cheese. Baked beans and spaghetti were acceptable and so easy to make.

The hardest thing was to make the effort to do anything at all but if I didn't I would just starve. Brian would bring me flasks of hot water to make up drinks before he went to the office each day but that was the extent of his culinary expertise. He also gave Mimi her breakfast and saw that Jamie was safely delivered to school.

Not one of the books had been read. I just idly turned the pages. They all seemed so full of enthusiasm and positive thoughts. I wondered if the authors had ever felt as I did. It is not easy to be positive when you are frightened and alone.

I didn't feel that I really ate any junk food – certainly not intentionally but I didn't feel any better. I had never smoked or drunk alcohol other than socially when I would much have preferred a coffee.

My symptoms were no better and I felt in limbo with someone or something needed to point me in the right direction. Two important events now occurred. I went to a homoeopath for the first time and I met Helen.

4

HOMOEOPATHY

Since visiting our new health food shop regularly the owners were helpful with practical advice to the many people new to the world of healthy eating and I learned a great deal from them. I informed them of the Consultant's advice to me and they immediately suggested that I visit a homoeopath who had just started a practice in our area. As he lived and practised on the south coast he only came for a few days each month but Dave and Moira were so certain that he could help me that on being given his name and telephone number I said that I would contact him with a view to seeing him.

This I did and in January 1985 kept my first appointment. He had a room in a local hotel which did seem rather incongruous for medical consultations and it was impossible not to compare the thick carpets, the highly polished furniture and the quiet with most medical waiting rooms. I was eventually called into the consulting room where I met a pleasant kindly gentleman. My first impression was that he seemed to have all the time in the world and he requested me to sit at his desk. I watched as he slowly filled his fountain pen with green ink, blotted it and tried it out before turning to me. Even though he was putting papers in order and settling at his desk, I felt sure that he was observing me keenly and was only too well aware of my nervousness as I clenched my clammy hands and waited for his attention.

He turned to me in a sort of quizzical way, half smiling with a hint of a questioning look with which I was to become familiar over the next few months and I could not contain any longer blurting out all that I had been told and my fears of now and the future and that in no way did I want to enter hospital, of how frightened and mistrustful I felt of conventional medicine and

21

how much I wanted him to help me. Half defiantly I told him that his friends from the health shop had said that he would be able to help me.

My relief was tremendous when in his quiet musical voice he told me that I certainly was not going to die and there was no need for the medical treatment suggested, so abhorrent to him was it on my description that he visibly winced. He assured me that he could help me and I believed him. Maybe it was because he was saying what I wanted him to say, but more than this it was the quiet authority and sense of confidence in his own ability that I instinctively recognised and knew that I could trust him to help me.

He cleverly eased my tensions by asking me about myself generally and about my family, what I knew of their lifestyles, ailments and occupations. It all seemed rather irrelevant to me but I was able to tell him as much as I could about grandparents, aunts, uncles and cousins.

It is amazing how difficult it is to remember details of a life but I tried as far as possible starting with my early ailments and life. I had had whooping cough when about three years old. From what our family doctor told my mother he had never seen a child have it as badly as I did and survive. I have vague memories of this illness and the fear of it, the panic it arose in me was to stay with me in some degree for always. Basically I was sturdy and healthy only having the childish ailments of measles and chicken pox mildly. I remembered the joy of playing with my father's chickens on the lawn and being content to stay with them in the pen, sitting with them in the dry dust and with our cat Blachie which were my first and faithful friends. Where we lived in a small group of houses we were surrounded by fields and what is now a nature reserve and farms and small holdings. Most of the time seemed long summers that I enjoyed with the few local children that I knew.

School started which I certainly did not enjoy with severe teachers and rules that I found pointless and I recall the relief from it when away with the catarrhal colds that I often had as a young child.

Life was simple with long nature rambles and rides on bicycles that all of us children had as a means of transport as well as for pleasure, and roller skating in the streets and skipping ropes and hop scotch, and of course swimming.

As I grew older I began to enjoy my education particularly geography and history and the new world of English literature and the power of weaving pictures with words that would assist in my career when I was older.

Cosmetic dentistry was a blight on my life from my early teens but it was the only alternative to dentures which filled me with horror, so I endured root fillings and jacket crowns and post crowns and two bridges. This was a great strain on me but at a young age it seemed important. Looking back I think I would have done the same thing but how much wiser it would have been if I had known more of dental and oral hygiene and taken more care of my lovely teeth and of course had I not eaten so many sweets and chocolate biscuits – but then we all have our weaknesses.

I enjoyed many sports including tennis and sailing and was proud of my climbing prowess on the Welsh mountains that were to be a constant joy to me, an appreciation of their grandeur taught me by my father and Uncle Bob who believed that education went beyond the schoolroom. My cousin Jan and myself were most fortunate in having fathers who taught us from an early age to appreciate all natural wonders in life.

When I was twenty three years old I had a mouth virus. I always remember first noticing it whilst on a family trip to the theatre with my Uncle Fred and Aunt Rose from America and biting succulent chocolates that tasted bitter and hurt my mouth. For weeks after that my mouth swelled and filled with puss and my oral consultant urged me to be admitted to hospital. This I declined but with his help he saved me from choking and after a few weeks of a diet of liquids and ice cream I recovered.

My only in-patient visit to hospital was to have Jamie when I was encouraged to have an epidural injection. This I did but always remember the fear I felt many hours afterwards when I still had no use in my legs. I was told that all would be well and I was only too glad to return home. From that time I have had lower back pain that I learned to live with greatly eased by constant walking and sitting on hard chairs.

It seemed to take a long time wading through my family history but the homoeopath listened attentively, making occasional notes.

He seemed satisfied that I had given him a clear picture of my life and explained that homoeopathy was different from conventional medicine. It was basically a natural healing process, providing remedies to assist the patient to regain health by stimulating the body's natural forces of recovery. It treated the patient rather than the disease and in no way tried to mask or suppress symptoms as these reflected the persons ability to overcome the illness.

My initial visit had taken well over an hour which left me feeling quite exhausted but in a better frame of mind than I had been in for months.

I eagerly awaited the arrival of the tablets which duly arrived and I was directed to take them under the tongue in a "clean" mouth that had not had anything in it for a least half an hour before or after taking the remedy. I was recommended to use *Nelsons* toothpaste which would not affect the efficacy of the remedy and at first I found this mild tasteless paste insipid after the normal positive flavoured toothpastes, but I soon became accustomed to it. During the course of treatment certain substances like eucalyptus and camphor were prohibited as they would nullify any curative effect.

Also taboo was coffee which was a dreadful blow to me. I had been recommended to use barleycup or dandelion coffee which I found vapid even when made strongly but I persevered and left my coffee jar untouched.

The tablets I took as directed did not have any adverse effect and from a mental point of view I certainly felt better until during a bath I felt definite lumps in my stomach that had not been there before. I soon began to panic but they did not give any pain so I endeavoured to contain my anxiety until my next appointment. This duly arrived and I was distressed to realise that on this occasion I would be seeing an assistant to the homoeopath that I had not met before. She seemed such a young person that I did not feel very confident. I told her about the lumps and she also felt them and confirmed their existence. She was calm and said that she would see that I had a consultation with the homoeopath on my next visit.

During the following month I tried to improve my diet as directed and ate whole fresh foods daily and cut out white bread and sugar which I replaced with wholemeal bread and demarara sugar. I still ate meat, fish and chicken as normal plus plenty of cheese with buttered crackers which was an easy but sustaining meal. I began to eat more fruit and thoroughly enjoyed the organic dates obtained from t he health shop and also figs.

As I liked salt I changed to sea salt as recommended as this contained many necessary minerals.

It was with much relief that I kept my second appointment with the homoeopath and he obviously knew of my anxieties from his assistant. His calming influence had an immediate effect on me as he explained that symptoms like these lumps were nothing to get alarmed about. They were the body's way of getting rid of illness and a good sign, and as I was in no pain from them he certainly did not show any concern. This was such a different way of thinking to orthodox medicine that it did take me some time to adjust to it, but it did make sense so I tried to follow his advice and not worry about the lumps.

He did not want me to worry about anything and seemed pleased that I was making such an effort to help myself in taking the tablets as he directed and that I was altering my diet to a more healthy one. I was surprised that he did not greatly stress diet and he did say that the body would sort out what it needed from the food given to it.

Again I went home greatly relieved with what I felt was sound and sensible advice even though alien to my orthodox medical upbringing, and it was a comfort to know that he was only a telephone call away should I wish to contact him for any reason.

Over the ensuing months I saw the homoeopath's assistant on a number of occasions and I soon realised that her youthful appearance in no way detracted from her competence and she always gave me her full concentration and it was with pleasure and confidence that I found that a particular appointment was to be with her. I shall ever be grateful that I had the help and support of these two people at a traumatic time of my life.

It was with some excitement that I realised that I was beginning to feel better and that my gynaecological symptoms were less pronounced. This greatly urged me to help myself more as I still felt that I could make myself well again if I only knew how. I still felt that diet was the key to everything and that surely the answer must lie in the books that I now had but had not properly read. I just knew that this was the right direction for me but that all my efforts were like a huge jigsaw scattered over a floor and somehow I had to find the correct pieces and put it all together.

5

HELEN

Meeting Helen was one of those million to one chances that came after I noticed a letter from her in our local newspaper. What interested me was that she had visited the Bristol Cancer Help Centre twice and was awaiting a third visit and wished to share her experiences with anyone wishing to learn more and she would inform them of how to visit Grove House.

Neither of us was fit but we began to correspond and then she telephoned me to ask me to visit her. After a few abortive arrangements due to ill health our plans came to fruition and one afternoon in the Spring of 1985 I drove to her home to spend an hour with her. She opened the door to me and I was completely taken aback at the figure before me. She looked so incredibly healthy and strong with a well rounded figure and fair English rose looks. Her radiant smile of welcome made me so glad that I had come. I followed her into her sunny sitting room that was bright with flowers and we sat down and looked at each other with interest and curiosity. There was never any strain, never an awkward moment, and we were soon exchanging details about each other. She had had breast cancer that had now spread to her bones. She had been told that her body was healthy but that her bones were rotten. This is why she looked so well.

She was interested in me and wanted to know how she could help. I told her that I wanted to become well by my own efforts and I felt that diet was the answer and that in a way I was sure that she could advise me. She told me that she had visited the Bristol Cancer Help Centre twice and that it was a wonderful place where you were pampered and given time to talk and therefore be helped and of course given healthy meals that you had not had to prepare. A visit to the centre would be most beneficial to me but I told her it was out of the question as I could not leave my young child and besides I did not feel well enough to go.

I had to admit that I had not really studied the book and when I said that I enjoyed tomatoes and potatoes she said that I certainly should not be eating these. With her encouragement I said that I would read the book with a view to starting the diet as directed. She was doubtful whether I would stick to it as she said it was difficult to prepare one meal for yourself and another for your family. She knew that she shouldn't eat meat but when she had a meal with her husband John she would enjoy a joint of meat with him. She also had milk in the weak tea that she drank even though milk was forbidden. I could tell that she was sceptical of my efforts which made me all the more keen to try.

She paused and looked round to see whether John could hear before leaning forward and whispering conspiratorially that she loathed brown rice. The hushed words contained much venom as she told me of her struggles to eat it at Bristol. She said it was so good for you but after endless chewing she could hardly swallow it. She looked at me half tearful and half defiant to measure my response to the outburst. Time hung in loaded stillness until I could contain my laughter no longer. As I told her that I felt exactly the same and that in no way did I believe anything so disliked could do either of us any good her kind face glowed and from that moment we became special friends.

In the future we laughed at my many disasters and exalted at my successes but we could always cheer each other with references to brown rice. Even now after many years I never see brown rice without thinking of our treasured times together.

She was a loving person and found great comfort in being hugged but due to the constant pain in her bones this was impossible so we touched ever so lightly but sincerely and just knowing that time was short made us unshy and able to express our caring for each other. Some of the new friendships made due to illness were very good.

Until the end of Helen's life we were constantly in touch with each other by telephone and occasional visits and I still have the letters that she wrote to me, always full of love and concern for me and at first full of hope for a new operation that she was to have or a new treatment until finally her courageous optimism accepted defeat.

In September 1985 her consultant implied that her life was nearing its end. She admitted to me how desperate she was and did not know what to do. As often as she was able, she spent time in her holiday caravan with John who was so supportive.

She visited Park Attwood Clinic for three weeks where she seemed happy and was helped. She had luxurious lavender oil baths and then relaxation in a warm bed. She was to have iscador injections and all the food was organic and vegetarian, much preferable to chemotherapy which she had discontinued at her request as it had made her ill. They seemed to do interesting things like painting and recognising that different sounds meant different things. Mmm is a warm sound so it brings love and D is a hard sound of earth so keeps us steady on the ground.

She had anthroposophical injections for pain instead of morphine which I was pleased to hear as I always felt that morphine was the final aid before the end.

Eventually Helen returned home and due to the condition of her bones had constant pain. She started chemotherapy again hoping that it would help her. She seemed so ill and I was glad when she said that she had been to Wasdale for a short holiday with John as I knew how much they loved the hills and lakes and how much he enjoyed fishing.

Gradually she got worse and John admitted to me that nothing had helped her. She pleaded with me to see a doctor or visit Bristol or Park Attwood as she was concerned about my thinness. Our friendship had been short but precious and she was the first person who really encouraged me to use my instincts and let them work for me. Through the months I had listened to advice from well intentioned people who wished earnestly to help me but I knew that none of this was for me. Helen's dear sweet face will always be with me and I feel I learned a lot that helped me through knowing her. She urged me to read *The Bristol Diet* book and I count this as the start of my recovery. At that dreadful time Helen was my lodestar, the one person who understood how I felt and she was the only sunshine in my frightened life. Our time together was always full of light and brightness and I welcomed her freely given love and encouragement to follow my feelings and fight for life in my chosen way. Her joyful memory will always shine brightly for me and be ever treasured.

6

THE BRISTOL DIET

The Bristol Diet was written by Dr. Alec Forbes who for twenty eight years had been a consultant physician in a Plymouth hospital. During this time he became more aware of the psychological and nutritional causes of disease. In 1980 he left the National Health Service to develop a working example of a new medical model for wholistic health care.

His interest in diet began in 1937 at Oxford University and I was fascinated to read that he tested all his diets out first by eating them himself before giving them to his patients; also that the diet was suitable to all conditions and to the general prevention of disease. This I found most encouraging as by now I had so many pains generally and aching in my joints that I felt my whole body needed detoxifying.

The recommended fast from food in the first instance I felt I could cope with. I decided that I would stay with mineral water as I liked it so much and that I would eat grapes, always the same type of grapes and in small amounts. This I really enjoyed and found most refreshing and it greatly lifted my spirits to be enjoying consuming something that should be doing me good. During this period I read the book completely and felt that this would be the basis for my recovery. I then read it again as I had decided that if I was to be on a diet for life then it must be one that would do me good and just as important one that would give me so much pleasure that I would never wish to return to my old ways of eating.

As I had never eaten large quantities of meat I felt that I would try a vegetarian diet as it was certainly recommended at this stage. As every meal had to be changed I decided to take it a stage at a time and to eliminate the things that I enjoyed most like chocolate and cakes and puddings last and the items that I felt I would not miss first, like meat, and particularly red meat as it contained a lot of growth hormones.

The meat meal that I enjoyed most was our weekly Sunday roast. So roast beef and yorkshire pudding with fresh vegetables and boiled and roast potatoes were on the menu for that first Sunday of my diet. I ate my usual meal complete with meat and savoured every mouthful of beef. I recalled the taste and texture with enjoyment knowing that it would be the last time that I would eat beef and I accepted this. On the following Sundays I did the same with tender fillet of lamb and thick loin pork and left chicken breasts until last with their complement of stuffing and sprouts. The following Sundays I had exactly the same meal with the meat gravy for flavour but without the meat. I found this acceptable without any meat substitute. With all of the meals that I was to change I always found that in doing the change gradually I allowed myself to become accustomed slowly and never moved on to the next change before I had mastered the first one. That way it was never a hit and miss affair but a definite and lasting change.

In one way this Sunday change was the hardest as it was the one meal that we ate together as a family and inevitably there were comments. My father had always eaten conventional meals and was most concerned that I was omitting the protein from my meal. These observations on a weekly basis that were tantamount to criticism did upset my equilibrium but I knew that it had to be coped with and that I was doing what was right for me. There was also the consolation that most of my meals were taken in a relay manner with people coming in at different times for meals and at midday on weekdays I was normally alone so there would be plenty of days when I could experiment unobserved.

Raw vegetables were recommended and this was something that I had never had in my life. If anything I probably over-cooked vegetables as I liked them to have a soft consistency. One day I decided to eat a raw meal and prepared some sprouts of which I was fond and grated some carrot. The change was far too drastic from my usual meal and after chewing and chewing in no way could I stomach raw sprouts and the carrot seemed so hard. That meal was a disaster and it was with some relief that I had tried it out when alone. I tried boiling my vegetables less and less until I was managing to eat them in a less than usual soggy consistency. Sometimes I put too little water in the saucepan and it boiled dry so I tended to stand over it with a fork prodding until it was just tender. Ten minutes was my minimum for fast cooking vegetables like broccoli and cauliflower and fifteen minutes maximum for sprouts and carrots that I did not enjoy if they were hard. Using less water in an endeavour to save the nutrients rather than tipping it away on straining the cooked meal resulted often in burned saucepans but I considered it all part of the change and bought myself a set of small saucepans solely for my own use on weekdays.

I had often had chops or steak or fish in the week and now that this was to be eliminated I did feel that I must try a substitute. At the rear of the book was what was to prove to be an invaluable list of what were and were not permitted to eat. In the health shop I was shown sesame, pumpkin and sunflower seeds. As these were permitted items I decided to try them in place of meat and fish. I had never seen any of these seeds before let alone eaten them so it was with much interest that I prepared my vegetables and on a side plate put a pile of sunflower seeds. I was delighted at the pleasure derived from this meal and it was so easy to prepare. The dark green pumpkin seeds I was a little hesitant over, but on another day tried these and again enjoyed them. The sesame seeds I did not like, not even in snack bars, biscuits or bread and I have never acquired a taste for them, but sunflower and pumpkin seeds were always to be found in jars on my pantry shelf after my initial tasting of them. Salt was not allowed but without it I found meals bland. As I had decided that it was important that I should enjoy my meals I decided not to put salt in the saucepan while cooking and only to use it sparingly at the table and always to use the sea salt sold in the health shop which contained necessary minerals for the body. This I found a satisfactory compromise.

Almond nuts had four stars against them which meant that they could be eaten plentifully. Normally I ate nuts at Christmas and only sparingly then, as Christmas cake and mince pies and boxes of chocolates were usually more to my taste. I bought a large amount from the local greengrocers and found the shells so hard that Brian patiently spent many an hour shelling them for me. He had a large mound of shells for a small jar of nuts. He also shelled walnuts, brazils and pecans which I tried for the first time and for which I developed quite a passion. From the start I never mixed any of my nuts or seeds, preferring to eat only one type at each meal. All of these meals I found enjoyable, making sure that I had a predominance of almonds as these were the most recommended. These meals were so strange to me at first that I was grateful to be able to experiment during the daytime when I was alone, but I soon became used to them and can truthfully say that I hardly missed meat at all. I still cooked meat or fish daily for Brian and the usual family Sunday roast, but I never felt the need for it and soon preferred my meals without the gravy, just having the nuts or seeds dry with a little salt. I was well pleased with my painless transition to a healthy cooked meal.

At this time I could find no supplier of organic foods so felt that I would do my best to have food as fresh as possible with as much variety as I could of the foods permitted that – most important – I enjoyed. I read of the adverse effects of artificial fertilisers and agricultural sprays, the latter which deposited toxic residues on the plants, which we ingest. I tried not to think about it but washed everything that I bought as thoroughly as possible.

It was with surprise that I read that certain cooking utensils could be bad for you. Aluminium or teflon coated utensils should not be used. An excess of aluminium could be taken in and apparently poisons were produced by heating teflon. I had never examined my saucepans before but on doing so found that they were a mixture of aluminium, teflon coated steel and stainless steel and that they were old. Stainless steel, iron or enamelled ware were the only types recommended so I visited the local market and purchased a variety of enamelled saucepans and three sieves of varying types to be used for washing vegetables.

It was a blow that coffee, tea and chocolate had to be given up. Apparently they contained caffeine which harmed various organs and functions. Herb teas and non-fluoridated water like bottled spring waters were suggested.

My lifetime habits were to be turned upside down. It seemed that all that I most enjoyed was forbidden. I continued to eat chocolate but concentrated on my drinks. Herb teas I found totally abhorrent. Not one flavour could I stomach without a shudder. Mineral water I now drank automatically and would never contemplate drinking a glass of tap water as I had done in the past. I had had my water tested and the visible results of contamination were horrific. It didn't even look clean. From then on I washed all fruit and vegetables in water from a purifier and also did this for cooking. I had always liked my tea and coffee hot, strong and sweet and to give this up was a wrench. I tried dandelion coffee but found this no substitute for coffee and decided to try all the "suitable" drinks that I could find.

I acquired a taste for Caro but missed the sweetners dreadfully. As I had decided to change my diet, from what I had read, for it to be effective and remain so, it had to be a lifetime commitment. I knew that I would have to enjoy it or I would never keep to it. I decided to try honey of which "very little" was permitted. I had never had honey in drinks before nor had to my knowledge eaten it. This I really enjoyed and made Caro a lovely drink. I also tried Luaka tea as it was reputed to be the purest available and with honey enjoyed this as long as it was strong and hot. I never even tried de-caffeinated coffee. I decided that as a healthy diet did not contain coffee at all I would not make life difficult by tempting myself with forbidden joys. When Luaka supplied de-caffeinated tea I felt cheered as I now had a variety of drinks that I enjoyed and were permitted and would do me good. To this day I still drink these same beverages together with Yannoh, Bambu and Maltfit for variety. My transition to a healthy and enjoyable liquid intake had been easy. Hot coffee made with whole milk and plenty of white sugar had for years been my favourite drink. Soya milk was recommended but in no way could I find this palatable so for a while I continued to make coffee as I liked it. I tried my other new drinks without milk at all and found these most surprisingly pleasant and refreshing and to my jaded appetite most appealing. After a while I also found that I did not need the drinks to be so strong and found the delicate flavours preferable to my usual coffee made with milk, which now seemed heavy and rather indigestible. I soon gave up milk in drinks totally and now shudder at the thought of drinking it.

Having eaten wholemeal bread for some time I was encouraged at the health shop to try some of their bread which was ordered specially and made with healthy ingredients. After my initiation to this bread I was rather hesitant to repeat the exercise but was given a slice of wholemeal bread to try at home. This I did and was pleasantly surprised by the cake-like texture and enjoyable flavour. I was soon converted to this bread and also took the opportunity to experiment with all the loaves that they sold. Their wholemeal bread became a favourite and I soon refused to eat anything else, always keeping a stock in my freezer for emergency use. This made excellent toast upon which I put butter, but not as liberally as previously, topped with a generous helping of marmalade. Like the Duke of York I was partial to Tiptree marmalade and over the years must have consumed tons of it. This was impossible to obtain in my home town but I had an arrangement with Rackhams of Birmingham who delivered it to me at intervals in large quantities. I knew that preserves were taboo but I enjoyed my breakfast so much that I continued with Tiptree to ensure an appetising meal. Some time later I was informed in the health shop that they had a new loaf that they thought I would enjoy called a cobber. It was a granary loaf of the type which was much recommended by Dr. Forbes, so I purchased an experimental one. It seemed incredibly grainy and chewy with an unusual flavour and over a few days I consumed the whole loaf. It had plenty of "body" and the usual wholemeal bread did not seem quite so appealing as before. I soon became addicted to the granary loaf and realised with surprise that in discontinuing my sliced white bread I had gone in stages from one extreme to the other and loved my new bread. I was also delighted to be eating so healthily with such relish.

Never had I eaten salads and the thought of giving up jam, cream, chocolate, cakes, scones, buns and biscuits was going to be hard to do. Lettuce, cress, radish and beet were all recommended but apart from the odd lettuce leaf I had never eaten these. It was with some misgiving that I prepared myself a salad which certainly looked colourful and appetising and I cut some of my granary bread with butter to complement the meal. I did not particularly enjoy it and decided that I would do this primarily on alternate days to give myself the perquisite of an enjoyable meal as encouragement. When beetroot was fresh in the greengrocers I bought some and boiled it and found this much more to my taste than the precooked variety that I had tried with vinegar.

In *The Bristol Diet* book sprouted grains were recommended as they were rich in vitamins and minerals and contained high quality protein. I purchased a sprouter but soon found the simple method of washing the seeds and putting them in a jam jar and covering the top with muslin far preferable. These I kept on the window ledge by the sink so that I did not forget to rinse them the required three times a day with cool water and it was fascinating watching them grow. I tried most of the seeds and beans in the health shop but all were forgotten after I had tasted the joys of lentils. They were time consuming to do as I liked to remove the outer shells after sprouting so that I was left with a pile of peach coloured lentils with white sprouts one quarter inch long. I found doing the lentils quite relaxing and therapeutic and the knowledge of their later consumption made it worth the effort.

As I never enjoyed any of the alternative spreads to butter and I could never tolerate any of the soya derivatives I always continued with butter but sparingly in the beginning.

I never missed the ham and tongue sandwiches that I usually ate or the generous slices of meat from the Sunday roast but omitting jam tarts and fruit pies with cream was much harder.

Perhaps it was fortunate that I was unwell as this diet certainly took up all my concentration and energy.

So that all my salad meals didn't seem the same I decided to have different items with a lettuce base as I soon acquired a taste for this. One day I would have lettuce with radish, another with beetroot, another with cress, another with watercress. I found this far preferable. I never had nuts in salads as I had these with my vegetables and I did like variety. One day a week I had free range eggs boiled with bread and butter with salt and pepper which made quite a change, but gradually I found that this seemed heavy and over many months I said goodbye to jam, cakes and pies without regret. I now had a salad every day and most important of all I enjoyed every mouthful.

I was now coming to the harder items to give up like custard made with full milk and treacle sponge, a favourite since childhood. I made my last pudding and savoured every mouthful, knowing that the ingredients were not doing me any good which did have a mental dampening effect but I did relish my last indulgence in this forbidden delight.

Chocolate was hard to give up. A lifetime consumption of mars bars, turkish delight, rolos, fudge and all that was bad for me plus chocolate biscuits would be hard to break. This was greatly helped by introducing carob chocolate and carob coated biscuits into my evening snack which was when I usually enjoyed a relaxing munch whilst watching television or glancing at the newspaper. Carob was no substitute for Cadbury but it was nutritious and I found it acceptable, but I never enjoyed it like real chocolate. Over many months I found that I did not need all the sweet foods that I had previously found so essential and I voluntarily gave up carob. I liked the wholemeal biscuits sold at the health shop made with non-animal ingredients and it was with surprise that I began to find the butter shortbread biscuits that I had eaten all my life far too sweet.

Just as I was never to enjoy brown rice, I found the same with boiled beans. Perhaps all the washing, soaking and rinsing I found incredibly slow and laborious and too much of a strain and my first soggy efforts hardly constituted an appetising meal. I experimented with the various coloured beans, peas and lentils, none of which were enjoyable so these were discarded in favour of complementing my vegetables with nuts and seeds.

Good health is something that most of us take for granted when we have got it. After losing mine and realising the hard struggle it would be to regain it I vowed never to take it for granted again. I would never accept it as my due but only as my reward for the effort I knew would be required to capture it again. My returning health was all the impetus that I needed to continue searching for the diet elixir that now eluded me. However long it was to take I would never yield until I found it, knowing that this was the only sure way to achieve optimum health.

Digesting *The Bristol Diet* had taken a long time but it had proved surprisingly edible and I knew this would be the basis of my future food pattern. Even then I felt it was the tip of the iceberg and that there was a lot more to learn and that I had yet to discover the perfect diet for me.

7

WILL TO LIVE

Corresponding with the commencement of my new lifestyle was the incentive and hope to live. This had temporarily left me but now returned in the first instance because of Brian's offer to purchase a holiday home for us in Criccieth. This had for many years been our second home and we felt we belonged there nearly as much as we did in the Midlands. The flat that we rented annually was one of a block of four and the ground floor one had now come on the market.

We made a visit during Easter of 1985, a lonely journey through the snow-capped mountains of the Cymru land to an almost empty resort that we had never seen so deserted. I was able now to walk along the promenade and was filled with pleasure to know that on this visit we had finalised our purchase of the flat and part of this special corner of Wales would now belong to us. I always feel that this was greatly instrumental in helping my mental attitude take a leap forward in contemplating the future times to be spent in our own holiday home. These dreams were realised many times and never can we journey to Criccieth without the tense excitement as we near our journeys end and make the final turn that gives us the picture always in my mind of Criccieth nestling beneath its Castle and the gentle curve of the bay and its long beach. I have a constant reminder of this scene painted specially for me by my friend Alan. We have now seen all Criccieth's moods. The heat of high summer and the swarms of scantily clad holiday makers, the grey angry seas of autumn when it was unsafe to venture onto the jetty for fear of being swept off and the clean dawning of spring when we would walk along the wide shingle beach with only sea sounds for company and the distant bleating of sheep on the mountain. I shall always be grateful to Brian for stretching our resources to their limits to help aid my recovery.

Another purchase – equally important – was that of a back support chair. For years I had found lower back pains aggravated by sitting for too long on easy chairs or settees and preferred the hard seated dining chairs. In my early fretful state I found the only comfort was to lie on the bed, but as this was a temporary respite I opted for the settee where I would lie many a dreary hour and from where I watched the woods at the rear of our home through the seasons and in some way drew comfort from their quiet greenery. Quite by chance I saw an advertisement for a back support chair. It looked most strange but the posture of the model was the position in which I felt most at ease. Brian thought it looked most odd but as he had some idea of how hard I was trying to help myself get well he agreed that we at least go and look at one. As soon as I sat on the chair I felt it was part of me. I never had a moments doubt that this would assist in my recovery and that it would be part of the jigsaw that had to be fitted together to make me completely well and whole again. We purchased a chair and came home and assembled it. It caused much amusement and most people were intrigued by it and had no idea how to sit on it and to me they looked as uncomfortable on it as they said they felt. Strangely, the only people who enjoyed sitting on it were Jamie's friends. All the children seemed just as content to sit on it as I was. Over the months it greatly eased my back pains and encouraged my general posture. These chairs were to be my Christmas and birthday gifts until I had four – three for our home so that I did not have to move chairs from one room to another and one for our holiday home. For many years these chairs have been part of me and one is taken on all of our holidays as a necessity. My chosen lifestyle is adhered to daily as far as possible and I know that this is why I am successful.

One of the great joys in my life had always been to be physically active. In my younger years I had run for sheer pleasure, revelling in my body's supple mobility as I would run in roads, parks, round the garden and the greatest pleasure of all, barefoot on the beach by the sea, hardly noticing the damp sand as I lightly sped along. The thrill of dinghy sailing was also associated with my early years and I was fortunate enough to have a number of friends who allowed me to "crew" for them. There is nothing quite like the lift of a boat when the wind is directly behind or the exhilaration of sitting out and trailing my hair in the sea as we glanced over the water. I loved the solitude of the mountains of North Wales and as a young child had climbed with my father, uncle Bob and Jan. Ingrained in me was an affinity with nature and the desire to be part of it and savour all its goodness, lying on sun-soaked grass under a brightly painted blue sky with only midsummer hum for company or climbing over rocks on a wild wind-swept beach beneath menacing scudding clouds. All of these I had been part of all my life and I wanted to be well enough to be part of them again.

As slowly I began to get better I decided to start to walk again which I had been unable to do, first round the garden which was a tremendous feat and the most important as it was the first step. My confidence had totally evaporated so I did this alone as I wanted no onlookers to witness my laboured walking. As I improved I wanted more than just the garden. I walked up the road but nerves and fright overcame me and I went back indoors, weak and perspiring and thankful for the sanctity of a quiet house. The next day I tried again and this time went the distance of two houses. Soon it was three and then four houses and then I walked right to the end of the road. This was an achievement and I was grateful that I lived in a quiet area where for the most part my efforts were undisturbed. At the end of the road I had to sit down on a convenient wall before starting for home and this was done in all weathers. I must have looked a strange sight sometimes sitting out in the rain.

This walk became my daily routine, always done first thing in the morning as soon as I was left alone and as I became stronger it was a pleasurable anticipation rather than the endurance test of my early efforts. As I sat at the end of the road I eyed the park opposite as to walk in it was to be my next hurdle. I looked at the nearest tree and the first time that I felt able walked to it. The park made me feel out in the country and a part of all that was good. I leaned against the tree, feeling the gnarled bark against my fingers and pressing strongly against my bones as I leaned against its strength. I looked up at the sky through its leaves and felt a surge of joy at my progress. I retraced my steps, stopping at the wall to rest before going home. Over the ensuing months I walked further and further. Using the trees as stopping points to rest, I felt like a bus stopping at all the stages but the important thing was I was making slow but sure progress. The trees became my friends; we knew each other well. I talked to them and felt them give me strength and encouragement as I leaned against them. I knew their moods and became aware of their annual changing cycle and rejoiced in their new spring birth and their mighty summer unfolding with high branches sweeping the sky with their dark greenery. Green had always been my favourite colour, my bridesmaid Trish had worn it and it was the colour of my "going away" outfit too. Some green had always been in my life at important times and all the park was green.

The momentous day came when I could walk all round the park. Of course some days were easier than others and the elements helped as well. Fog I had always hated; it created ethereal pictures of moisture on my trees and plants but I did not like the clinging damp fingers that reached to my bones. The rain I revelled in as I sploshed along, usually alone when it was torrential. There was a certain pleasure feeling the rain running off my face down my neck and I would often return quite soaked, but with an immediate change of clothes I never caught cold. I looked upon rain as a friend and welcomed its varied music, from the insistent drum when it was heavy to the light drizzle that gave me most pleasure with its soft gentle touch on my face and the smell of damp on the grass. I always walked on the grass and never the paths and kept close to the trees. I always felt so much better after walking in the rain. The crisp snow of winter with the glinting sun making sparkling crystal patterns as it covered all my green made a bright crunchy world for my walks and I welcomed all the seasons. Summer, when everyone complained of heat but me, I loved most. It was never too hot for me and the feel of the sun warmed me completely and lightened my heart even though a bright blue sky looked gaudy and unreal. It came that hardly a day of the year my walk was missed and the park played a vital part in my recovery. It was there when I needed it. Even now after a weeks holiday my first day home is highlighted with a walk in the park when I renew myself with all its pleasures.

A few friends stopped calling when I became ill and unable to join in their fun times which made me sad. Gwen, who was like an aunt-sister-friend never stopped coming to see me and was so dependable that she was a rod to lean on. She was the only person with whom I left Jamie when he was a baby and I trusted her absolutely and with gratitude I still value her help given to me when I needed it.

Gwen came to see me twice weekly with total dependability. She was the only person who saw me preparing my meals as she always came during the morning. She would sit and watch me preparing a variety of vegetables, usually with plenty of carrots and she must over a long period of time have watched me shell hundreds of nuts. I would offer her some of what I was preparing but she always declined. She was curious about my diet and as a "conventional" eater admitted she would not want to eat my diet. She never criticised or tried to dissuade me from my chosen way and took the view that if I enjoyed it that was my prerogative to eat as I chose. I much appreciated her attitude as she was in a position to undermine the small amount of confidence that I had at that time. Over the years she was to mention how much fitter I looked and how much better I was and commented on the length of time since I had been in bed too ill to come down to her. At first this was noted in weeks, then months and now years. I know she is surprised as she was one of the few people who saw me at my worst moments.

Sheila, whose son Colin grew up with Jamie and at one time lived close by was the other person who offered to help in any way. She would have had Jamie for me and this was a great comfort to know that he had a family he could go to should the need arise. As I became well she told me how ill she and her husband Phil thought I used to look. I was so thankful that they never told me that at the time.

As some of my friends deserted me so I felt let down with my association with people that I had met through the Church. This made me turn from God for a while until I realised that He would never forsake me and I had allowed unsympathetic members of his Church to cloud my judgement. Now I do not belong to any Church but feel closer to God than ever before. I say my prayers daily and with joy in the quiet of my home and when I am out walking free of all pain. He has guided me to have the strength to work out my own salvation and helps me in all things. I try to live a Christian life and most of all to be true to myself.

All of these things helped me to survive in the early critical days but most of all I felt it was my own determination to live. Of course I wanted to live for my father, husband and child but I was honest enough from the beginning to know that I wanted to live for myself. Life is our most precious possession and seeing mine slipping away when I had so many good things to live for was unendurable. Helen was the only person to encourage me to go it alone and this was a tremendous help, but even without her I feel that I would have succeeded. Maybe being an only child and used to spending long hours alone with only my thoughts for company had enabled me to think for myself and always to question other people's ideas that they knew best for me. As I get older I feel that I know best for myself and the greatest truth of this is my continued improved health. I accepted total responsibility for all my decisions with complete confidence and have never doubted that I did the right thing for me. I have never felt the need for compromise and have always gone my own way through life however unconventionally. This total belief in myself was my greatest asset as I started the long haul out of the abyss that I was in. I truly never found it difficult. I was just able to see things as they were and how through lifestyle, stress and tragic losses I had come to my sorry state of health. Never shall I sink so low again. I recognise all the danger signals that shout a warning to me on bad days – and I do have bad days – and immediately put my own mental improvement plans into action. It gives great confidence to be able to recognise the start of a downward spiral and to climb out before sinking too deep into the mire. My strong will and determination were my best allies.

Getting well is the hardest task that I have ever undertaken and after monthly visits to my homoeopath in August 1985 he signed me off as I seemed well. I remember clearly asking him whether he thought his medicines or my diet had cured me. He took the view what did it matter as long as I was well. It mattered to me a great deal as although undoubtedly he had helped me – mentally from our first meeting – at that time I did feel that I had done a great deal to cure myself.

Although free from gynaecological pain and symptoms I hardly felt strong or completely well. I knew that I was pointed in the right direction but still had a lot to learn and was to a large extent groping in the dark. I decided to explore all avenues to help me become strong and glean all knowledge that I could. I was still convinced that I had not found the total curative diet for me yet and was determined to do this.

8

SEARCH FOR DIET

In my search I read every book and article and watched television programmes in my quest for complete knowledge in devising my own health regime. Many books I found too "way out" and not at all suitable whilst others had the odd item that I found useful. I gradually sifted out what would be helpful and learned a great deal during the process.

One of the first books that I read which was of great interest was *Raw Energy* by Leslie and Susannah Kenton. Leslie Kenton was the Health and Beauty Editor of *Harpers and Queen* and I was familiar with her face from the newspapers. She always seemed full of energy and so incredibly young that I felt she must have some original ideas about diet. Having been brought up on the idea that at least one cooked meal a day was necessary it was intriguing to find a book in the main totally opposite to this. The idea was to eat seventy five per cent raw food grown on healthy soil and eaten fresh. The book gives real life instances of proof that raw food can be life giving. The Swiss physician Max Bircher-Benner was one of the great European pioneers of nutritional science. He came upon the potential of uncooked foods when he was ill and unable to eat. His wife, peeling apples for dinner one day, slipped a small piece of the raw fruit between his lips. He found it pleasant and unlike all the other food that had been offered to him - digestible. Several days and many well chewed apples later he had completely recovered.

As a doctor he was soon afterwards called upon to treat a patient who was apparently unable to digest anything. Discussing this case with a colleague he was told that in 500 BC Pythagoras wrote of curing a similar condition by giving nothing but mashed raw fruit, a little honey and goats milk. He was rather sceptical as he had been taught that raw foods are difficult to cope with if you have an ailing digestive system. He decided to try Pythagoras' remedy and the next day tests showed that the patient had digested the food properly. A digestive system that could not handle cooked food thrived on raw food. Spurred on by his patient's remarkable return to health Max Bircher-Benner began to investigate the special properties of 'living food' as he called them and to use them to treat other illnesses. Regardless of the type or seriousness of the illness his living food treatments were an enormous success. The clinic which he founded in Zurich in 1897 continues to be one of the most highly respected centres for healing in the world. He also insisted that a patient be treated as a whole person – with the end in mind not only of curing illness but also of making that person as wholly well as possible. He found that a diet high in uncooked foods played a central role in this self-realising, self-healing process.

The German physician Max Gerson started to experiment with his diet in an endeavour to cure migraine. First he tried milk, reasoning that since it was perfect for babies it might heal him and be easy to digest, but on a milk diet he felt sicker than ever. He then turrned to fruit. Like Max Bircher-Benner he started with apples and cautiously extended this basic regime to include other fruits. His headaches stayed away except when he added new items that disagreed with him. He ate fresh fruit and vegetables for the rest of his life.

I was excited to read of his book *A Cancer Therapy*. He believed that the starting point for all illness, cancer included, is an imbalance of sodium and potassium, usually too much sodium and too little potassium. If the balance is corrected by eating potassium-rich foods, which invigorate and cleanse the body because they improve respiration at the cellular level, this also mobilised the white blood cells which fight and destroy cancer cells.

After reading many fascinating instances of recovery it did seem obvious that the mainly processed foods generally eaten posed appalling dangers to human health. The answer was that human health was related to wholeness and freshness of foods that we consumed and that the only way to achieve a high level of health was to adhere to a diet rich in uncooked foods.

The biogenic way of life was also mentioned which was something that I had never heard of. It was based upon the writings of the Essenes, a monastic sect that flourished on the shores of the

Dead Sea at the time of Christ. These ancient texts have quite specific instructions about health and healing and stress and the use of fasting and raw foods to achieve potent mental, physical and spiritual health. Biogenic practitioners regard all illness as the manifestation of a single disease; disharmony. The biogenic way of eating consists of about forty per cent fruit, because fruit is ideal for ridding the body of its own wastes and thirty per cent raw vegetables. Grains, dried fruits, dairy products, seeds and nuts made up the rest.

After many years of research the Linus Pauling Institute in California found that a raw food diet – fresh apples, pears, tomatoes, carrots, wheat grass, sunflower seeds and bananas – was found to have cancer preventing properties equal to those of a normal diet plus massive amounts of extra vitamin C. Vegetable fibre had also been shown to be protective against certain kinds of cancer, and specific vegetables – brussel sprouts, cabbage, cauliflower and broccoli contained compounds which had been shown to lessen the effect of cancer causing agents.

Leslie and Susannah Kenton's book introduced me to previously unheard of enzymes. They consider these to be probably the most important health-giving factors of plants and these are completely destroyed by cooking.

Enzymes are the essential triggers for every living thing. There are tens of thousands of them working away in the human body – some 50,000 in the liver alone - breaking down food and assimilating it, building new tissue and repairing it, and manufacturing more so that the vital work can continue. Apparently many practitioners believe that the enzymes in raw foods are important because they help support the body's own enzyme systems. Each food, they say, contains just the enzymes and co-factors (vitamins or minerals which are linked to enzymes) needed to help break down that particular food. When these are destroyed by cooking or processing, our body has to make more of its own digestive enzymes to digest properly and assimilate them. By ensuring that your body has an outside supply of enzymes, these practitioners claim, you should be able to live longer, look more youthful and stay healthier.

I was interested to learn that when seeds are sprouted enzymes which had been dormant now become active. Sprouts have many times more than the nutritional efficiency of the seeds from which they grow and provide more nutrients ounce for ounce than any other natural food known. Enzyme activity in plants is never so intense as at the early stage of sprouting. It was gratifying to know that the sprouts that I found so enjoyable were also doing me so much good. From now on the subtle energies of enzymes I would treat with respect.

Looking back I am relieved that *Raw Energy* was the first of the many books that I was to read in my search for the perfect diet. This book was so in accord with what I was already trying to do and seemed to complement perfectly all that I had read in *The Bristol Diet*. Plenty of fruit was fine by me. Admittedly my fruit had been that of the obvious English housewives purchase - apples, pears and bananas. As the seasons changed I looked forward to experimenting, but in the first instance I intended to continue with my raw daily salad meal with as many interesting permitted and enjoyable variations as I could find.

Up until now my cooked food had not been satisfactory but the idea of a steamer seemed the perfect solution to the choice of soggy or burned vegetables. Searching for a steamer in my home town was not easy and the only shop that stocked them only had an aluminium one which I knew was unsuitable. Eventually a local shop purchased an enamel one made in Poland which ended all my cooking problems and changed my whole appetite where cooked meals were needed. Instantly I noticed how different the food tasted. The flavour magnified and the texture was crisp. At first it seemed strange but I soon became used to it and now would never consider cooking in any other way. Fortunately I purchased two steamers as they have now gone off the market. After many years of constant use they look rather dilapidated but are considered vital to my get-well programme and I cannot contemplate being without them.

One book that attracted my attention, probably because it was written by a person local to me was *Curing Arthritis* by Margaret Hills. Like most unwell people I seemed to have a variety of ailments including aching bones and stiffness in my joints so fortunately I decided to read this little gem. I always call it my serendipity book because of the meal that is a regular firm favourite with me to this day that I found in its fascinating pages. Honey was recommended as it was packed with natural vitamins, minerals and trace elements, plus many more including iron which was in greater quantity in darker honeys.

Molasses was recommended but in my ignorance I had never heard of it, but as it was described as a "wonder food" and full of valuable food elements I thought it worth investigation. When sugar cane is crushed, the juice that comes out is sweet, but as good nutritionally as is other fruit juice. It is concentrated by boiling and the refined sugar crystallises and is removed by spinning. Three or more boilings and spinnings are carried out and the remaining syrup, which now contains all the sugar cane goodness in a concentrated form, but minus most of the sugar is "black strap molasses". I was also amazed to learn that 10 per cent of molasses was made up of iron, copper, calcium, chromium, phosphorus, potassium, magnesium, zinc and a variety of trace elements. With all those minerals in its natural state it just had to be good. I tried every make of molasses that I could find and my palate found Appleford's crude black strap molasses by far the most enjoyable.

Margaret Hills put porridge oats at the top of her list for a breakfast meal, it being a natural food and one of the most wholesome and well balanced ones available. I had never eaten porridge before but its easy preparation made it attractive.

Ever since I had used a sterilising unit for Jamie's meals when he was a baby at the heart of a cold winter I had had aching finger joints which I definitely attributed to constant immersion in cold water. Up until this time my fingers had been supple no doubt helped by consistent use of a typewriter. Also since I became ill I had aching knees plus general aching bones, particularly in my chest.

Over the ensuing months I tried every porridge that I could find and soon felt as much a connoisseur of this as I was of water. By far my favourite was Mornflake organic oats and I always made my porridge with Volvic mineral water rather thicker than is suggested as this gave a more substantial meal. This I topped with a generous spoonful of molasses that soon melted to give a rich brown coating to my creamy porridge. This not only looked good it tasted so too. As I wanted to give it a proper trial I had this every morning and after a few weeks felt the pains in my bones gradually decreasing. Eventually they went altogether and after many years I only get pains in my bones if I have to go out in the cold for too long and get chilled. This meal was also excellent for

being a bowel regulator and so easily digested. When I felt quite
well in my bones I alternated the porridge with my much loved
wholemeal toast and marmalade and felt no ill effects.

In my search for the ideal diet for me it was inevitable that I
would come across many variations of what was an ideal diet. One
of these was Macrobiotics. It is a Greek word and its translation is
"great life". The leader of the International Macrobiotic
Movement was Michio Kushi whose book *The Cancer Prevention Diet*
makes fascinating reading. Macrobiotics is a revival of Japanese
traditional medicine, a means of balancing the yin and yang or
acid and alkaline qualities of the food we eat. On a deeper level it
was a discipline, a way of living, a means to restore the health and
harmony of mind, spirit and body. It was a recognition of the
unity of man, nature and the universe. It was about food for the
soul, food to nourish physically, spiritually and emotionally. By
eating only natural foods a person becomes more aware of his
body and of nature and of the closeness of the two. By creating
balance in foods we eat, we in turn create balance in our lives,
particularly in our attitudes.

Macrobiotics was the way of eating practised by Zen Buddhists
and was rediscovered by a Japanese named George Ohsawa. He
stated that physical and mental disorder comes from a disordered
unnatural way of eating. Fifty to sixty per cent of the diet is brown
rice or other cereals. Most of the rest is vegetables and pulses.
Animal fats, meat of any kind, dairy products, milk, cheese, butter
and yoghurt should be avoided. Michio Kushi was also opposed to
vegetables of the solanacae family - potatoes, aubergines, tomatoes; no refined sugar and no salt, no honey or other sugars. No
fruit. No tea. No coffee. Only Chinese bancha tea was permitted.
A typical days eating for getting well would be porridge for breakfast, wholemeal bread and sugar free marmalade; for lunch, vegetable soup, protein, usually in the form of a soya derivative such
as tofu and bancha tea; for dinner, pressure cooked rice and vegetables and perhaps stewed fruit. A macrobiotic diet does not
advocate raw vegetables and salads, but vegetables are only lightly
cooked. In general a macrobiotic diet for a healthy person would
mainly consist of rice, vegetables, pulses and seaweed. Rice, the
"soul" food would form the basis of the diet. Grains should

account for over 50 per cent, legumes 10 per cent, animal foods 5 per cent, soup 5 per cent and desserts, fruit and nuts 5 per cent. Occasionally a little fish or meat may be eaten.

Another yin yang principle was to eat "seasonal" food native to your country. In a hot yang climate, yin foods should be eaten to cool you and in a cold yin climate, yang foods should be eaten to warm you.

Michio Kushi states that vitamins exist naturally in whole foods and such pills taken as a supplement to regular food produce a chaotic effect on our body's metabolism.

He also advocated that fresh fruit be eaten only a few times a week, preferably cooked or naturally dried provided that they grew in the local climatic zone. He also states that fruit juice was generally too concentrated for regular use. All flour products are excessively mucus-producing which should always be remembered and ice cold foods and drinks including ice cream were not recommended.

I was interested to learn that dietary practice according to macrobiotics was the way of eating that flourished from before the time of Homer to the Renaissance. It was the diet the Buddha ate under the Tree of Enlightenment and that Jesus shared with his disciples at the Last Supper. It was the diet that helped Moses free his people from bondage and that sustained the Pilgrims upon their arrival in the New World. Most of all it was a way of life followed by ordinary people throughout history.

Certain items stated by Michio Kushi differed from other books that I had read. He advocates food being pressure cooked and *The Bristol Diet* states exactly the opposite. These differences I found a challenge as I was not merely trying to copy any one person, but to gain from their knowledge and experience to found my own diet. One thing that all of these people had in common was total dedication to their chosen diet and way of life. In this I was in perfect agreement and accord, never once had I become disheartened at all the time and effort involved and never ever disillusioned because I had my continuing improving health to encourage me to carry on searching. Because of my dislike of rice and also millet that I tried I knew that this diet in its entirety would not be for me, but I did extract valuable information that I would put to use in my own diet. The intriguingly named bancha tea so much recommended to this day I have not tried. Of my two local health shops one had not heard of it and the other could not obtain it. I shall try it if ever the opportunity arises.

Better Sight Without Glasses by Harry Benjamin was first published in 1929 and my father had a well read copy of the twenty second impression of 1943. As I had always had excellent sight and in fact was extremely long sighted which I had always found most useful I was not enthusiastic when he offered me his copy to read. He urged me to read it as Mr. Benjamin's panacea for all eye problems was based on diet. Since I had become ill my eyes had felt tired and strained so in my open-minded continuing thirst for knowledge I opened this unheard of volume. When I realised that it was based on his own personal experiences of rapidly failing sight in spite of wearing enormously powerful glasses to eventually being able to discard the use of them altogether I sensed that here was a true story of great courage and conviction.

Mr. Benjamin stated that we ate in order to live but many people had lost sight of this sole purpose of food and instead of looking upon eating as a necessary function to be performed with the same object as breathing and sleeping, it had come to be regarded as a means of gratifying our desires for the nice things of life - not of merely satisfying our hunger. The chief criterion of its value was not that it should contain the elements most necessary for the health of our bodies, but that it should please our palates and our senses generally.

I thought for a moment. Although I had enjoyed my bad diet just as I was now thoroughly enjoying the experience of eating real food, I had never been a person who lived to eat and most definitely ate to live. This I found tremendously important and this made it comparatively easy to adjust without too many regrets. Chocolate I now would never think of eating and the family Sunday lunch that I prepared with traditional roast meat was of no interest to me and when I approached the matter my feelings were that this type of meal was now abhorrent to me. I would view my meal of lightly steamed vegetables and nuts with relief that that was what I was to enjoy. Even steamed puddings and custard were now items of the past. As I educated myself on the ways of a good diet I accepted all prohibitions if I was to get well. I was never tempted to backslide because I never wanted to.

Mr. Benjamin brought attention to the neglect of natural

foods, such as fresh fruits, salads, green vegetables, root vegetables, dried fruits, dairy products and honey and nuts, and where green vegetables were used they were invariably boiled, thus denuding them of their valuable salts and health-giving properties.

These items he felt made the best possible basis for a sensible healthy diet, and all who valued their health, or wished to regain it, should see to it that these foods were well represented in their daily diet.

Meat or fish should be eaten sparingly and as fresh as possible.

Cereals were also necessary but likewise were sufficient if eaten once a day and genuine wholemeal bread was most suitable.

He stated that the best start to a day should be a fruit meal of fresh or dried fruit with fresh cold milk. This seemed most strange to me as by now I was more than content with my choice of toast or porridge.

Lunch or evening meal should be a salad, consisting of lettuce, celery, tomatoes, cucumber, watercress and grated raw carrot together with wholemeal bread, butter and cream cheese. If a salad dressing was required it should be lemon juice and pure olive oil. A second course could be stewed prunes and cream.

The third meal could be anything within reason, such as meat, fish or egg with steamed vegetables. Potatoes when used should always be baked in their jackets. Dessert could be dried fruit and nuts, baked apple or egg and milk custard.

He stipulated never to use condiments or drink with meals and cut down tea and coffee to a minimum and always eat the freshest food possible and nothing tinned or smoked. Bread should be eaten only once a day and if a drink of tea was wanted it must be weak and without sugar. For certain medical conditions he states that coffee should not be drunk nor alcohol. Neither should pickles or sauces be consumed. Although any fresh fruit in season was recommended bananas never were even though he does not give a reason for this omission.

For some eye conditions he also recommended cleansing the system of toxic matter by a thorough course of eliminative treatment. The best way to begin was to undertake a fast for from three to five or six days on orange juice or water or both and then begin the diet.

All of this I found most fascinating and exciting as in so many ways it followed the recommendations of *The Bristol Diet.*The idea of a fruit breakfast stood out in startling contrast as I had always believed that a good meal was the best start to a day with fruit only after main meals or as healthy snacks between meals. Apart from this I felt most heartened as it dawned on me that whatever illness I had it could be improved with good diet and that this was the key and the only key to permanent good health. All the time I felt that I was learning so much and yet there was still such a lot more to learn.

I shall always be grateful to my father for drawing my attention to this book's existence and over the years I have borrowed it from him on many occasions to refresh my memory on certain points. I view its battered dust cover with affection for it has served me as a true friend.

As a young teenager I spent many happy hours on my bicycle, often with my contemporaries as it was the normal mode of transport to school when we would share our secrets in conspiratorial whispers in the way of young people who were friends. Most of our pastimes were spent outside but all of us loved the cinema. There were many local picture houses as they were called where the double billed programmes changed halfway through the week and together with the forthcoming attractions and news made an excellent diversion from homework during the evenings. We would eagerly cycle to the various cinemas when we knew that the bill boards would be changed to see whether any of our special favourite film stars would be appearing. I was no exception in this passion for films and like most of my girl friends longed to emulate the glamourous film stars with their exotic lifestyles.

This liking for films and interest in the sophisticated world of the stars had always remained with me so when browsing along the library shelves the book *The Beverly Hills Diet* by Judy Mazel claimed my attention partly due to its title and partly by the picture of a golden pineapple on the dust wrapper. I expected it to be stories of particular film stars who spent their lives on a diet of pineapples. On flicking through the pages I could find no obvious stories of film stars, but as fruit was mentioned a great deal I decided to read it.

This book promised to its faithful followers a lifetime of thinness which appeared to be the aim of most Americans. Having no desire to become thinner I mused that if I reversed everything that I read I would probably put on weight. I started to read Judy

Mazel's book. From the beginning you felt her reaching out to help you in the open way that I associated with Americans generally. Her book contained a fascinating new concept of eating that was alien to my orthodox diet and explained how she had gained health and slimness by experimenting on herself until she had a tailor-made diet to suit her lifestyle. As this was exactly what I was endeavouring to do myself I read on and was rewarded with so much knowledge that I found logical and good sense. Judy Mazel was transparently sincere and totally enthusiastic that her technique of conscious combining of food would work for everyone and to me her secret formula seemed meals of simplicity. She talked of prehistoric man not eating breakfast, lunch or dinner but who would eat a meal of berries, kill an animal and eat it, then find nuts and chew them. She talked of "mono meals" where she ate only one food at a time. She found that the digestive system worked better this way and it was obvious to me that this made sense as the body would not have to work as hard digesting one type of food as it would with the usual mixture.

Judy Mazel's diet of conscious combining was based on putting foods together that digested together – foods that worked together. This was the way not to get fat and to achieve good health and a high energy level.

I decided to forget her obsession with thinness but to concentrate on her sound ideas that health, energy and well-being hinge on the quality of the nutrients our bodies processed.

Like *The Bristol Diet* she starts with a thorough cleansing of the body with a commencing diet solely of fruit then gradually introduces other foods correctly combined.

It was fascinating to learn that the stomach was about the size of a small grapefruit as I had always imagined it for some reason to be much larger. Fruit was the mainstay of Judy Mazel's diet and she began almost every day with it. This did interest me as Harry Benjamin had suggested this same meal but as yet I had not tried it.

Most of the books that I had read so far ran on parallel lines in that they all advocated fresh food that was produced as naturally as possible with plenty of organic vegetables if obtainable but none had suggested "mono meals". All my life I had never been greatly impressed by a lengthy menu, but was more than satisfied with one main meal followed by something gorgeously gooey.

I decided to try "mono meals"

My first meal was jacket potatoes with plenty of butter and salt and nothing else. My plate looked quite strange but I enjoyed the meal and did find it completely satisfying. For an uncooked meal I had a large plate of bread and butter which I also liked despite the omission of a generous portion of jam that would have been my preference. One day I had a meal of almond nuts, another day my favourite pecans, and another day walnuts. These meals were as promised satisfying but seemed peculiar to me and I didn't dare think what my family would say if I gave them any of these items singly as a total meal. I also tried a meal of Judy Mazel's highly rated pineapple which was her symbol. This was surprisingly satisfying but so strange for a meal. All of these seemed so unusual. Her rule that could not be broken was to remember only to eat proteins with other proteins and fats, carbohydrates only with other carbohydrates and fats and always to eat fruit alone. After a lifetime of ending meals often with fruit pies or tarts with cream or custard it all seemed like a foreign language and yet there was no doubting Judy Mazel's sincerity and total commitment to her lifestyle. I could certainly understand that when she was invited to social functions she checked with her hostess first to see if there was anything suitable on the menu for her and if not asked to bring her own food. Many times I put down her book as being so way out and yet the more I thought about it the more it made sense. As I read through the book I learned to like Judy Mazel's very much for her zest for life and determination to live her life her way.

Reading as many varied books as I could obtain on health and diet had given me a wide knowledge that I had not had before. I had learned so much that I felt I could incorporate this knowledge in a lifestyle plan of my own. Gaining this information and storing it in my mind for future use had taken many months and I still had not found the missing link that would make it all come together. My school motto had been "to strive, to seek, to find and not to yield" and I remembered this on the days when I yearned to put my body totally in order. Yet when I paused and thought I realised that the yawning chasm of frightening blackness that had so often in the past threatened to engulf me was now gone for ever. In spite of my experiments with diet which did not always work I had found many new and for me novel ideas that did work and I was getting better and I had started to put on weight. It was with renewed confidence that I turned away from the terrifying days of constant ill health and fear of an early death which were receding for ever and that is when I found the book that was to transform my whole life.

9

FOOD COMBINING

F *ood Combining For Health* by Doris Grant and Jean Joice didn't look anything startling or different from all the other books that I had read when I found it one day sitting patiently on its library shelf waiting for me. The words "don't mix foods that fight"! on the cover reminded me of Judy Mazel's conscious combining and when I saw the foreword by Sir John Mills I thought maybe that this was an English version of the American book. My weakness where film stars were concerned and the intriguing information that the book was based on the Hay System prompted me to bring the book home for what on earth was the Hay System. The smell of hay I certainly found earthily intoxicating and always had since in my childhood I had been fortunate to spend holidays on a friend's farm and grew to find pleasure in the daily farm aromas.

Reading Sir John Mills words immediately dispelled any ideas that the Hay diet was remotely connected with farming but what was important was his obvious enthusiasm for a diet that had not only cured him of a duodenal ulcer in 1942 but that he had lived in fitness ever since entirely due to his continuing with the diet.

William Howard Hay was born in Pennsylvania USA in 1866 and in March 1891 graduated from the University of New York as a Doctor. For the next sixteen years he practised medicine and surgery until his own health failed. Fearing that his life was in jeopardy he was inspired to treat his own symptoms. He did this by eating 'only such things as he believed were intended by nature as food for man, taking them in natural form and in quantities no greater than seemed necessary for his present need'. To the great astonishment of his doctors his symptoms gradually disappeared and at the end of three months he felt fitter and stronger than he had done for many years. This experience, he wrote, deepened the conviction that had been growing over the past sixteen years that medicine was on the wrong track; it was merely fussing with the end results of a condition instead of attempting to remove the cause. His own illness had opened his eyes to the possibility of treating disease along dietary lines.

Dr. Hay's System consisted of five important rules:-
1. Starches and sugars should not be eaten with proteins and acid fruits at the same meal.
2. Vegetables, salads and fruits should form the major part of the diet.
3. Proteins, starches and fats should be eaten in small quantities.
4. Only whole grain and unprocessed starches should be used and all refined processed foods should be taboo – in particular, white flour and sugar and all foods made with them, and highly processed fats such as margarine.
5. An interval of at least four to four and a half hours should elapse between meals of different character.

Proteins require an acid medium for digestion. When animal proteins enter into the stomach this stimulates the production of hydrochloric acid which activates the enzyme pepsin, whose function is the splitting and digesting of the proteins. This action in the stomach can only take place in a wholly acid medium.

Carbohydrates require an alkaline medium for digestion. This is initiated in the mouth by action of the enzyme ptyalin, which splits the starches into lower forms before entrance into the small intestine where their further reduction and main digestion takes place. As the whole process of starch digestion depends on its proper initiation in the mouth, all starchy foods must be thoroughly chewed, otherwise the small intestine, although alkaline in all its secretions, cannot complete what the ptyalin started higher up in the tract.

Dr. Hay states for optimum health and heightened resistance to disease the diet should, ideally, consist of alkaline-forming foods and acid-forming foods in the ratio approximately of four to one, which, when metabolised, will produce a corresponding ratio in the body.

The easiest way to do this is to arrange the day's meals so that animal protein is eaten only once a day, cereal starches are eaten only once a day and the third meal contains neither but consists only of fruit with milk or yoghurt.

Alkali-forming foods comprise all vegetables (including potatoes if cooked in their skins and the skins are eaten), all salads, all fresh fruits (except plums and cranberries), almonds and milk.

Acid-forming foods comprise all animal proteins such as meat, fish, shell-fish, eggs, cheese, poultry, nuts (except almonds), all the starch foods such as grains, bread and flour and other foods made from cereal starches and sugars.

Small correctly combined meals are better digested and therefore more satisfying than large orthodox meals; it is not the amount of food that counts but the amount that is properly digested, absorbed and metabolised by the body. This was particularly pleasing news to me as though undoubtedly my appetite was slowly improving as I became well again, it was hardly the eager appetite of a healthy person so it was gratifying to know that one small correct meal would be most beneficial. What was even more exciting for me to read were Dr. Hay's words that paradoxically, compatible eating was equally helpful to people who were under weight! Both overweight and underweight conditions were due to abnormal states of body chemistry. Therefore, just as compatible eating produced a steady loss of weight for those who were overweight, so would it also produce a gradual building up of weight for those who were too thin. As at the onset of my illness my weight had dropped to under seven stones this was tremendously cheering news as I considered a satisfactory weight for me would be eight and a half stones as I had always been slimly built. This system of eating was first and foremost a normalising regime. This fact clearly indicated that nature works continually to restore us to the ideal in weight, stature, health, efficiency and everything else.

Dr. Hay maintained that we only needed protein in small quantities and that all the elements for human health could be supplied by fruits, greens, roots and milk. He contended that meat, eggs and even cereal foods were not essential and in large quantities they could over-stimulate and over-burden the metabolism. He also stressed that complex dishes should be avoided and that the best meals were composed of simple dishes of unprocessed foods and limited to two or three items.

He also regarded breakfast as a superfluous meal but if needed should be a light meal of fresh fruit. This would provide the alkaline meal which was so important. A well flavoured apple was most recommended. Apples - this reminded me of Dr. Max Bircher-Benner and his apple cure. Simple meals – this reminded me of Judy

Mazel's 'mono meals'. All of these experts in the field that I so desperately needed followed similar lines with fresh real food predominating and eaten in simplicity.

The Hay Diet I knew was the key to the life giving diet that I must devise for myself. It was the final and most important piece of my life jigsaw to which I now had all the pieces and only I could fit them together correctly as only I knew of my personal needs. For many months now I had been eating correct food but not correctly combined. It all seemed so obvious to me now but without *Food Combining For Health* my health and happiness would still be in jeopardy.

10

MY LIFETIME DIET

Inow looked forward with total confidence to assuming
responsibility for my dietary habits and the enormity of my
decision I accepted. I only had to look into a mirror to see
that I was no longer etoilated but had the healthy patina
gained over the past months of eating correct foods even
though not correctly combined.

Parallel with devising my new diet I also decided to encompass a
general lifestyle that would compliment it and give my body every
encouragement to regain not only good health but to give me
boundless energy and joy of life such as often seen in young children, but which gradually fades as the years encroach. Life is the
most wondrous thing that we have and I commenced my mammoth
task sure in the knowledge that I would succeed.

Initially I checked all the books that I had read and notes that I
had made and decided to eliminate all the foods that were unsuitable. Out of the recesses of my memory I recalled a childhood
friend of mine Roz telling me that she had to enter hospital for a
digestive related operation after which she would be on a strict diet.
Just before entering hospital she gave herself the forbidden but
greatly relished treat of a large plate of chips. This last defiant ges-
ture allowed her to accept its omission for the future. At the time
this had greatly amused me but I could see the logic of it and decided to do the same.

Of the deadly nightshade family which were unsuitable for cancer
patients I enjoyed potatoes and tomatoes. Following my friend's lead
I duly steamed two large potatoes in their jackets, cut them in half
and liberally spread butter on them topped with salt. I savoured
every delicious mouthful of my mono meal, chewing slowly to make
every mouthful count and to obtain total satisfaction from my meal.

This I also did with tomatoes that evening. Firm ripe English tomatoes at the height of their season were a rich red, resting in firm slices on a bed of lettuce. No meals could have been more enjoyed. With no regret I have never eaten potatoes or tomatoes since. My life was far more important than a short titillation of the palate.

Also reputed to be carcinogenic that I enjoyed were parsnips and celery. Parsnips I had enjoyed since childhood mixed with melted butter and whipped into a cream as only my mother could do. A celery stick dipped in salt after every crunchy bite was another salad favourite, but both of these I eradicated in the same way as the tomatoes and potatoes.

Rhubarb and plums were not recommended due to their high acid content. Now these were harder to give up as I prided myself on my pastry making and took great pleasure in making pies in the rhubarb season from rhubarb grown in my garden. Piping hot from the oven coated with caster sugar and doused in thick milky custard, it is my idea of edible paradise. I admit I succumbed to eating a whole rhubarb and a whole plum pie in this way before turning away from them forever.

Bananas, I decided to exclude from my diet, if for no other reason than that Harry Benjamin, in his book *Better Sight Without Glasses* recommends that they should not be eaten. I have never considered bananas as a fruit in the accepted sense, as to me they are always rather heavy and more like a meal. They conjured up memories of childhood meals shared with my mother on returning home from school and being cut into rings and made into sandwiches. The delicious bread that we had was baked into a shape that looked like two loaves stuck together, a thick golden-brown crust on the one side, like two miniature humps. My mother would break it in the centre to reveal the feather-light soft bread. We would each have two rounds cut from the centre of the loaf liberally spread with the loose butter of delicious flavour, obtained from our corner shop. These would be generously filled with banana rings and consumed with much enjoyment. This delicacy was certainly not permitted due to bad combining and if Harry Benjamen thought it best not to eat bananas I accepted his wise words.

Having eradicated all that was undesirable, I turned to the wealth of foods that were recommended as being beneficial to restoring and maintaining good health. There were three important rules that I had to keep. The first was that no food that was carcinogenic should ever be eaten. The second was that the diet be as simple as possible, bearing in mind the mono meals that Judy Mazel had used to such success. The final rule was that all meals were properly combined at all times.

I had read books on vitamins, minerals, calories, and the importance of watching weight. I decided to follow none of these. This diet was to be loads and loads of fun. A diet for life, not a mathematical exercise, which I would hate, and I am sure anyone else would too. I decided that if I ate all the good things in their freshest condition, raw or lightly cooked, I couldn't really go wrong, particularly if I used the guidelines I have just mentioned. I would be guided by my instincts – they had always worked well for me in the past and I knew they would now. I decided to let my body tell me what it wanted, and if I listened I would soon know whether I was giving it the right foods. Not just how something tasted in my mouth but how my body felt after it (the food) had been eaten. If I was eating the correct foods my body would feel perfectly satisfied after a meal and yet light. This diet has taken over a year to evolve before I was totally satisfied that this was the best diet for me within the scope of the foods available. This is a good basis for anyone's diet. From all the differing books that I have read, I realise that a good diet is good for a healthy person, imperative for a sick person, and whatever is wrong with you, it can only get better if your diet is good. I took the view that there was just no way that I could go wrong. I had got to get better. I was going to get better, and this is how I did it.

I think it is easiest to start off first thing in the morning. When I got up, I suppose like most people, I enjoyed a drink. For the first few months I just had mineral water when I was on my get well diet, and this was fine. Mineral water is the best that you can ever have, but as I got better I wanted more variety. I am the sort of person who likes variety. I would hate to have the same thing day in, day out. I never drank fruit juices. I considered that fruit juice should only be consumed in its natural state – and that is in fruit.

So, of all the drinks that were available I decided that I would start the day with my favourite drink, and this made good sense. This was Caro, made of course with mineral water- not hot, not cold, but pleasantly warm - so that the generous teaspoon of honey I put in it would melt. By this time, I considered myself a connoisseur of honey. I had systematically tried every honey that was available in the health shop and had acquired a taste for the lightly flavoured clear honeys. Of them all, Rowses Australian Honey was easily my favourite and must surely be the nectar of the gods. I did not use honey primarily as a sweetener, but as a highly nutritious, easily digestible food which was quickly absorbed into the body.

To obtain the maximum benefit from all food eaten it must be enjoyed to the ultimate degree. Time must be allowed to savour the delights of all that I chose to be edible. All meals should be taken in quiet, relaxed surroundings with the only thought in mind to appreciate the delights of every morsel. First thing in the morning this is not easy. There is the inevitable rush to get to the office and school on time and the first meal of the day in our home is usually a hurried affair. Nevertheless, I do my best, taking the view that if you try your hardest, you can never be counted as a failure.

As the palate becomes accustomed to natural, unprocessed foods it does not desire strong flavours nor the extremes of hot and cold and appreciates everything consumed to be of a moderate temperature and tranquilly flavoured. I savoured my cup of Caro with pleasure. It was important, the first thing to be consumed for approximately ten hours, so it was something to be looked forward to and greatly enjoyed. No more the hot, strong drinks of the past – my body didn't want shocks anymore – it wanted to be treated with consideration and respect. I drank my warm sweet drink slowly savouring each mouthful and feeling its warmth course through my body as I swallowed the aromatic liquid. It was the perfect way for me to start any day.

Breakfast now consisted always of fresh fruit. There was an abundant variety available throughout the year, so much pleasure was given to my morning menu. The great plus of a fruit breakfast is the negligible preparation time. Fruit is a marvellous way to start the day. I would never ever return to my heavier breakfast of bygone days.

Dr. Max Bircher-Benner, who found out himself the importance and health-giving qualities of apples was right – there is never a better way to start the day than with a well flavoured apple. What can beat, in the autumn the flavour of an English Cox's Orange apple. This I often had alone, sometimes with blackberries, freshly picked in the autumn in the country – a perfect pastime – something to do when a summer is ending in the mellow warmth of the autumn. What a restful way it is to spend a few hours in the countryside, and what joy to eat the fruits of your labour throughout the year. These freeze well and it is also free food. Blackberries and apple are an ideal combination, and one that I thoroughly enjoy. In the summer, when I can't get Cox's Orange apples, I substitute these with Golden

Delicious, which don't have a tang, but nevertheless are pleasing, and with these I have my own, organic home-grown raspberries. The first raspberries are ready at the end of June. Pick them in the evening surrounded by their rich aroma, still warm from the day's sun. They need not be washed, it is not necessary. Just keep them in a cool place until the next day when they will be eaten, full of goodness with an apple from my own apple tree with a flavour reminiscent of a sweet Coxe's apple, ripened in late September. I had the pleasure and interest in watching the first brave spurts spring into life through to summer when its leafy glory partially concealed the ripening fruit that was so delicious and essential to good health. There is a satisfying sense of fulfilment in growing your own food. I combined raspberries and blackberries with apple because both of those berry fruits I found too tangy alone, but eaten with an apple were delicious. I never ate a fruit that needed sweetening. I felt that things should be eaten as naturally as possible, and this was a perfect way to eat my raspberries.

Of course the list of fruits is endless, but one soon finds out what one likes best. In the summer, when we are satiated with choice, my favourites, I think, must be peaches; beautifully purple-ripe with their soft white down coats. Two average sized peaches make a perfect meal for me. Bite into them, into their golden blonde plush interiors, squeeze them gently in your mouth, and feel the liquid flow down your throat. Absolute ecstasy! What could be better? Peaches, I always feel go hand in hand with nectarines as they are available at the same time. They are a similar fruit, but have a harder, glossier skin and a slightly firmer texture inside and with a paler golden colour, but are equally delicious. Squashy English strawberries, with their glorious gaudy red colour, invite you to eat them. A plateful can be quickly devoured, but only eat them when they are fully ripe. You learn to choose fruit that's ripe. If it is under-ripe it is bitter and doesn't do you any good at all, and if it is over-ripe it could ferment. We don't really want to get drunk on our breakfast! Strawberries, with their heavy marshmallow texture can be compared with nothing. They are just heavenly.

Large black succulent glossy cherries are something else that I adore. As the season for these fruits is fleeting they must be enjoyed while you can get them. I must admit to discarding my staple diet of apples when I have these treats for such a short time.

Apricots are particularly recommended for cancer patients, and these I find gorgeous. They are eaten best when they are a deep yellow with a slight give to them; this means they are ripe and full of juice, more chewy than nectarines and peaches, but nevertheless an absolute delight to eat when they can be obtained.

Many fruits, of course, we can now get all the year round including all varieties of grapes – I personally like the large black ones with pale pink interiors, maybe because they look so good or because they are so large, or maybe because they just taste so good. Fully ripe plump green grapes with their cold green exterior and opaque centres can be surprisingly sweet and make a perfect meal. There is a large variety of pears – my particular favourite being the squat Packam pears. Choose these when they are a lemony yellow and just ready to eat and have just a slight give in them when you touch them. Firm rounded Nashi pears whose invitingly yellow skins hide an amazingly white icy textured fruit that has a distinct flavour and are loaded with juice, are a joy to eat. Often if you buy something that isn't fully ripe you find that when it has ripened it may be bruised and damaged, whereas if you buy something that is just ready to eat you know exactly what it's condition is, and of course you only want to eat anything in pristine condition. The fruit that I find has the most life-giving vitality in it is pineapple. This isn't quite so easy to choose, but it should be a golden colour, not lemon nor green nor brown, but a sunny golden colour. It should be firm to the touch without being hard, never soft – this means it's damaged or over ripe. If you smell the base of it it should smell fragrantly sweet, and if the leaves in the top can be gently moved then this is perfect. Slice it in half – I found half a pineapple was adequate for one meal. Cut it into sections – it's golden colour invites you. The first mouthful is full of glorious juice. You can actually feel the energy going into your body. Nothing gives you instant vitality like a pineapple. What the secret of them is I do not know. Maybe it is because it is packed with bromelain, an enzyme which activates the hydrochloric acid in the stomach and helps to break down protein. It is also believed to soothe internal inflammation, accelerate tissue repair, stimulate hormone production and clear away mucus in the gut. The enzymes in pineapple also boost dull, tired skin and so become a beautifier externally as well as internally. Whatever it is it certainly works. If I ever feel jaded generally there is nothing like a pineapple to pick me up.

I only think of eating dried fruits when I can't get fresh ones, and as of course I can always get such a large variety of fresh fruit, then I don't really need to buy dried fruits. I just have them if I want a change. My favourite of these without doubt are the Hunza apricots. These are nothing like ordinary apricots, in fact they don't look attractive at all. To me they always resemble a small walnut and in fact in colour look something like this: ruffled and crinkled. Soak them overnight in mineral water, not heated, just cold water poured over them. The following morning they will have swelled, and to put one into one's mouth is to experience a flavour like nothing else. It is incredibly sweet, syrupy sweet, but absolutely exquisite. These were part of the staple diet of the Hunza, a race reputed to be the fittest in the world or one of the fittest in the world, whose longevity was legendary . I assume that they would eat them fresh, not dry, and of course I've never been able to eat a fresh one – I've never had one. I hope one day to try them, but in the meantime, their dried variety is perfection.

Prunes are an easily obtained dried fruit, and soaked overnight are nothing like the custard and prunes variety that we used to have as children. Never buy pitted fruit. Lots of nutrients are in the kernels so soak all dried fruit in its entirety. Any goodness seeping from the kernel will be an added treat to a healthy energising meal. By themselves they have a sweet flavour. The hard crinkled coats become soft and plushy as you sink your teeth into them.

I never eat grapefruit and personally never recommend anything with such an acid taste. Thinking about it makes ones teeth jangle. I never eat anything that I need to put sugar with.

Melons to me don't have much flavour, and I like fruit to have flavour, so I rarely eat those. The intriguingly shaped carambula or star-fruit, to me, are like a frozen melon in texture, so I just eat these occasionally to add to variety.

The fruits that I have mentioned are my first favourites, and there is an infinite variety of breakfast choices.

I never mixed my fruits – other than the apple – with blackberry or raspberry, and that was really to make the raspberry and the blackberry edible, rather than wishing to combine. Eat each fruit alone. Never have any more fruit throughout the day. Fruit is only to be taken as breakfast. Remember this rule and you'll never go wrong. Your body will serve you well because you're giving it the best start to the day, cleansing, highly nutritious and the easiest of all foods to digest.

Always purchase organic fruit whenever possible and let everything you eat be as close to nature as it can be.

Mid-morning most people enjoy a break with a drink and a snack. Omit the snack but enjoy a drink with mineral water or one of the many health drinks. I have always thought the drinks labelled "coffee substitute" a misnomer as to my palate they in no way resemble coffee but are enjoyable in their own right each with its own subtle flavour. Savour it with warmed mineral water and of course I like mine with honey. This mid-morning drink is the final part of the daily body cleansing and keeps the digestive system up-to-date and moving swiftly which is vital for good health.

Remember to keep the gap between meals of different types to enable correct digestion and the recommended four hours interval is an excellent guide. Lunch or dinner can be interchangeable according to personal inclination or convenience. For a cooked meal always use stainless steel or enamelware and every item of cooked food that I eat I steam. This helps retain full flavour and nutrients and nothing is thrown away. My investment in an enamel steamer was essential as previously I only had conventional saucepans. An oven is now obsolete as all cooked meals should ideally be steamed for as short a time as is enjoyable. I am unable to fancy raw vegetables but have gradually reduced the cooking time until I now like them slightly crunchy and therefore more health-giving and as a bonus for the cook so much time is saved by cooking for short duration. All food should be as fresh as possible and where obtainable organic. This is more expensive but far more tasty.

Fortunately I have a local supermarket whose range of healthy organic fresh foods is constantly increasing. There is a great pleasure in growing your own food and investing in a tasty apple tree and a few soft fruit bushes is an easy way to start. Vegetables and salad foods require more time for good crops but growing them is a fascinating way of obtaining health food.

For my cooked meal I would always endeavour to eat seasonable vegetables as this gives variety but always with plenty of carrots as I consider them a most important health-giving vegetable as well as being sweetly delicious partnered with another vegetable. The myth that carrots help you to see in the dark is true as they have an abundance of the nutrient beta carotene which can be readily converted to vitamin A by the body . Vitamin A is essential for vision in dim light and low levels of this vitamin is known to cause night blindness. During the growing season the amount of beta carotene increases so mature deep orange coloured carrots have far more goodness than young ones. Again I observe the rule of simple meals but without the rigidly strict 'mono meal'. I never have more than two different types of vegetable at one meal and one is usually carrots. The important protein I have from nuts and seeds and there is enough variety for a different choice for each day of the week. Nuts are full of protein and oil imperative for good health and completely natural, particularly when bought in their protective shells. There is no need to worry about additives and preservatives. They are free of all these unnatural substances. Participation of their enjoyment only adds to the fun of shelling them. A large variety of nuts is always available at Christmas time but not to me locally for the whole of the year. If you search as I did you can usually find a shop willing to help and I quite unexpectedly found Jenny who has a greengrocers and supplies me with nuts in shells all the year round. Most health shops sell the shelled variety but whenever possible always shell your own.

In summer there is the greatest choice and sweet garden peas cooked for a few minutes with sliced carrots accompanied by freshly shelled walnuts is an appetising and satisfying meal. This is the only time in the whole day that I have salt and this is not added in cooking but a small amount of fresh sea salt obtainable in health shops I feel is necessary to health as it contains many valuable minerals. It also gives the meal added flavour.

Garden runner beans I find easy to grow and if planted in an area of a mixture of two feet of garden compost well rotted and soil with a layer of peat on top this should produce a healthy bean. Beans steamed with diced carrots and eaten with almond nuts is a tasty easy summer meal. Never cook nuts. Eat them raw and as fresh as possible.

Rich green calabrese florets and slices of carrots blend in harmony with almonds. Almonds are the only alkaline nut and are much recommended by Dr. Alec Forbes. I find them delectable and they always find their way into my midday meals twice a week. They are also rich in oil and essential minerals like zinc, magnesium and potassium and have the highest amount of vitamin E of all nuts.

Broad beans are satisfying and of such a positive flavour that eaten with a plate of brazil nuts make a sustaining meal.

Pecan nuts have a delicate flavour and when chewed a creamy

texture. These partner cauliflower well to make a different type of meal. I never eat cauliflower with any other vegetables, only the chosen protein food.

Hazel nuts are happy eaten with small whole carrots and swede in winter or alternatively with whole carrots and turnips. The carrots and nuts give a lift to the milder root vegetable taste.

Filberts and distinctive mid-winter sprouts full of flavour after seasonable frost and carrots cut into rings is a favourite meal of mine.

Sunflower seeds I can eat by the handful but also make a colourful meal with purple tipped broccoli and carrots and add variety to my nut meals.

Spring cabbage that melts in my mouth or the firmer savoy I relish and with my faithful carrots partner well with pumpkin seeds.

All of these meals are most attractive which initially is important to the enjoyment of a meal. All items can be interchanged to suit personal preferences but I always eat only one protein item at a time. This aids digestion and gives meals more individuality. All meals should be eaten in relaxed surroundings with lots of time for absorption of the food for regaining and maintaining perfect health. Take a few deep breaths before the meal. If possible sit by a window with a view of your garden and nothing is more relaxing than being surrounded by trees of all sizes and colours. Every bite must count and be thoroughly chewed. There should be no more sitting in restaurants with friends talking animatedly whilst stabbing at pieces of food and swallowing them half chewed. I have been guilty of this myself countless times and if I pause to think and am honest I doubt I noticed what I was eating at all and now know that it did not give me maximum benefit. I had learned that the most perfect meal eaten hurriedly or whilst under stress would be better left until a quiet time when the food would be taken as it should be, with plenty of time for full enjoyment. Whilst eating, the meal should be the only item that you are aware of and your whole person should be given to savouring it. What a delightful way to regain health.

All of these meals are incredibly simple to prepare and can be cooked in minutes. Like most things in life the simplest is often the best and I find these meals sufficiently varied and satisfying to be more than adequate as a main meal of the day. Correct diet also gives correct weight. There is no need ever to count calories. Just eat enough to satisfy your appetite and this can only be done if you concentrate on eating properly and listening to your body. It will tell you when it is satisfied. Most people would find this diet ideal for losing weight but as an under-weight person this is not what I wanted, but I trusted the diet and my instincts and gradually my weight increased by one stone which is an appreciable amount. This of course in turn gave me confidence to continue and over the months I gradually accept-ed these more unusual meals as normal for me and was sur-prised to realise that I no longer wanted the average normal diet and turned only to my new one. This gave me all the life force I needed plus the joy of eating appetising meals, every mouthful of which helped me to return to good health. I had never been a great meat eater and unless it had been lean and tender had invariably pushed it to the side of my plate and ignored it. Now that I had this alternative of nuts and seeds that I welcomed, my protein intake was far greater, but without the heavy full feeling that was evident after a conventional meat and two vegetable meal. Although feeling satisfied my body was light and I liked this as I wanted to be active. As an extra bonus my mind was also more alert. This diet was a perfect body balancer.

Remember, never drink with meals. Have a mid-afternoon drink as mid-morning. Never snack between meals. Your body wants a rest and you will savour meals far more with an edge to your appetite.

What by far is the most important meal of the day is a salad. This must be taken daily to aid, regain and then retain optimum health. Without this I do not feel good health is possible. I do not mean the cessation of illness but the glowing feeling of good health that makes every second of every day a joy to live in and isn't that what we are all aiming for?

At first I just put all the salad foods that I could find together which made a rather dauntingly large meal that totally overcame me, so after much thought I decided on the rule yet again of simplicity and balance and variety. This was far preferable and as with my cooked meals, would enable me to have a weeks variety so that each meal would be different from the previous day and therefore aid satisfaction of the meal. In addition was the impor-tance of giving my body a chance to assimilate a larger variety of nutritional food in a semi-mono style to aid digestion.

It is imperative that all food be as fresh as possible and kept cool either in the salad drawer of a refrigerator or a cool pantry. Living in an older type house I am fortunate to have the latter which I find invaluable for storing my supply of fresh fruit. I usually do the bulk of my shopping only once a week as like most people I lead a busy life and could not possibly shop daily for my food, nor would I wish to do so. Good food is essential to my life but not to the point of dominating my existence. Find the best shops that you can. Most greengrocers will welcome a good regular customer. Even in my local supermarket I find that it is possible to request certain items and if possible they will be obtained for me. Organic food is becoming easier to obtain and I have no difficulty in finding the necessary unorthodox foods that make up my diet.

Never over wash saladings. Garden produce hardly wash at all. You don't want to wash away the goodness. If limp that means no life and all food should be crisp and snappy and full of life force. An added attraction of this diet is the bright colour of meals that makes them so inviting. No more pushing away a plate of dull uninviting food. This diet cries out to be savoured. Each mouthful should be anticipated eagerly and then chewed thoroughly; all concentration should be on the fun of eating, knowing that each mouthful is aiding good health and that every morsel tastes simply superb.

I never use condiments of any kind and certainly not salad creams or dressings. I want to taste the salad food and nothing else. Good wholesome food needs no dressing and only dubious foods need camouflage. Just have clean food washed in the minimum of cold water and shaken or lightly patted dry.

There are many jokes about salads consisting of soggy lettuce but the basis of all my salad meals is lettuce and certainly not the soggy variety. There are many types and each one at a separate meal gives a totally different meal. My first favourite is the English round lettuce with tender leaves. This with sprouted orange lentils makes an attractive dish and all of my salads are eaten with granary bread, the more grain the better and spread with unsalted butter. Choose a pale coloured butter as this will be the most natural. Crusty bread with soft interior and delicious aroma makes a satisfying meal. Remember the rule "simplicity is best" which aids digestion and therefore you can eat as much as you like to be satisfied without feeling bloated and any weight loss or gain needed will soon be achieved. I like to alternate my salads with what I call a "green" meal, usually with cress or watercress that is rich in iron and good for the body and maybe because it is my favourite colour I always enjoy it. The softness of watercress goes well with the crunchiness of iceberg lettuce and gives crisp mouthfuls of goodness.

Salad cress can be kept in the container that it is growing in and washed and sliced across for use just before eating. This makes it a living food that is ideal with Webbs Wonderful lettuce.

The dwarf Cos lettuce Little Gem with rich green leaves and elongated heart with delicate yellow leaves is crisp and sweet and available all the year round. Eaten with bright red small whole Scarlet Globe radishes makes a special lettuce dish.

Lollo Rosso lettuce with frilled red tinged leaves is crisp and originated in Italy. It mates perfectly with beetroot in texture and colour and makes another original salad meal.

Lamb's lettuce is available in the winter and has small velvety leaves and a mild delicate flavour. I never think of this as lettuce as it looks so unlike the normal ones and I actually use it to accompany another conventional type like English round lettuce or for a totally different look, flavour and texture with the crisper Tom Thumb.

Batavia is a large crisp head type lettuce originating from France with light green leaves. This always seems to be cool and joins admirably with crisp celery that I have for the occasional treat.

Quattro Stagioni is an Italian round lettuce with dimpled glossy leaves. It is looser leaved than normal green round lettuce yet firm and tender. This goes well with French breakfast, an elongated white radish with pink tipped bottoms.

Feuille de Chene lettuce is distinguished by deep bronze, serrated leaves. It has a mild but distinctive flavour and I find it a pleasure to eat alone during the summer months with granary bread spread with pale salt free butter. Alternatively this can be accompanied by Red Pearl radishes whose deep rich colour hides a firm thick white interior.

Pride of place as my favourite salad dish has to be a fresh summer round lettuce arrayed with beautifully coloured pale orange sprouted lentils with their firm white tails. The flavour of sprouted lentils has to be sampled to be appreciated as there is nothing to compare with them. They are well worth the few days spent on sprouting them in an empty jar and leaving in the kitchen to watch as miraculously they change from hard brown bits to orange edible loveliness. They – like all sprouted beans, peas and seeds – are a living food and nutritionally are incomparable and should be included in every salad diet.

As you will see limp miserable lettuce I threw out of the window an age ago and replaced it with these exciting varieties to give the base of perfect meals for well over a week. It is all so attractive to view, a pleasure to eat and so easily digested and so good for you. And did you know that lettuce aids relaxation?

These are my main meals of the day and I feel they are good for everyone and believe me I love them all and participate in them with eagerness and savour them with relish. Each so different from the previous one that I have infinitely more variety than when I ate a conventional diet. I would never want to alter my diet now, I find it perfect for me.

These meals can be enjoyed all the year round. Food does not have to he heated to give internal warmth. My salads are a fit meal for anyone at any time and their goodness can be enjoyed equally on a cold mid-winter day sitting by a warm fire as on a height of summer day on a picnic, savoured whilst sitting on a river bank or hidden in the folds of the mountains of Wales.

Never underestimate the value of a salad. It is as equally important as my other two main meals and it is a meal that I will never forego as to do so would endanger good health – something never to be allowed to happen at any price. Learn to love a salad; it will reward you a hundred fold with its life force of good health.

By now it will be obvious how much importance I put on to simplicity and this cannot be over-emphasised. Over the months I have also learned to recognise the foods that my body enjoys and the ones it prefers me to leave alone. Always listen to your body. It will always tell you what it wants. I love my greengrocery shopping and when in the shop or store surrounded by a bevy o f choice I do what I call "body dowsing". Just walk around, take your time, pick up the fruit, feel the texture lightly, smell it. Your body will let you know if it is pleased and its instincts are always right. Do as your body advises and you will never go wrong. Now I find it hard to go past any greengrocers without taking a peep inside to see if they have anything new for me to try out.

When I say that your body will tell you what it wants I don't

73

mean the unnatural craving for coffee or chocolate etc. These are signs that the body is out of balance. I know this from my own experiences. If I feel jaded then my palate is also and demands oversweet foods. I immediately go on a days cleansing of the systems toxins and I will quickly return to correct bodily balance and harmony when real wholesome foods are again asked for. Let the right food give you health and you will wonder how you survived so long without it. You will feel wonderful and ready to face the world in total fitness.

My food day ends with a drink, usually Yannoh, Maltfit or Dandelion coffee compound made with mineral water and honey, warming and mellow and the ideal precursor to sleep. I am pleasantly tired and content that I do my best to help keep my body as it should be, full of brimming good health and vitality.

This is the diet that I followed for many months and gradually I became more and more well and I felt that I had found the basic secret of a good diet balanced in all the necessary nutrients which would help regain health from any illness.

My gynaecological symptoms and pains had disappeared and I felt so much stronger. My pallid skin was now a healthy colour and my dull lank hair was now growing strong and firm with a rich gloss that had been lost for many years. All of this was surely proof that I had been right in following my instincts and giving my body what it asked for.

Having found the basis for good health I wanted to continue to improve on it. Because I was determined to find my own way to return to health did not mean that I had a closed mind to any further advice and help. On the contrary I was constantly enquiring of people about their own diets, particularly if they felt anything was beneficial to them but for the most part I found most people just ate conventional meals without questioning the quality of them and if they felt unwell it was so easy to visit a doctor and take a few pills.

I did feel at this time that I needed more stamina and in the dim recesses of my mind I recalled something mentioned in *The Bristol Diet* book by Dr. Alec Forbes. I found the relevant passage which stated that he had been a vegetarian for a long time and knew that he took a nutritionally correct diet, but after seven years was getting weak muscularly and was also quite thin because his muscles were wasting. He visited a Dr. Kelly in America who stated that whilst some types of people who only ate vegetables remained in good health other types of people needed quite a lot of meat to stay well. Dr. Forbes remembered that when he ate a different diet whilst on holiday that contained meat he felt more vigorous but that this strength soon fell away when he returned to a strict vegetarian diet. He gradually started to eat meat, eggs and fish in small amounts and found that he gained weight and became more muscular and had the ability to swim longer and longer distances. This made him feel that not everybody could be vegetarian.

I pondered long on this as by now eating any form of meat was alien to me, not only for my strong views on eating animals but the fact that the meat available today has usually been carefully bred, fed and treated with hormones to make it fat. It is not the lean healthy meat of an animal that lives free and has to be caught before it can be eaten.

Chicken and turkey had been the only animal meats that I had ever enjoyed, so I decided to try a breast chicken portion to see if it made any difference to me. I steamed it well and teamed it with cauliflower florets and with a small amount of sea salt cautiously tried it. After so long the texture seemed so strange but I persevered. Immediately the meat meal was so much heavier than what I was used to but I decided to try this out once a week for a month to see if it made any difference. I was surprised to feel that it did and that bodily I did feel stronger for longer periods on the day of the chicken meal and also the following day. I overcame my abhorrence of eating animals and now also eat turkey as well as chicken but only ever once a week. I am fortunate in having Mario, who supplies me with the most delicious turkey and chicken breasts, who is kind enough to contact me when he has received a supply. I never ate carrots with chicken it just didn't appeal and I cannot stress the importance of making a meal look attractive so that its consumption only adds to the joy of the meal. I always enjoyed only one vegetable with chicken. As well as cauliflower, broad and runner beans in season, winter sprouts taste crisp and crunchy with the added bite of some frost on them. I also liked chicken with spring and savoy cabbage, so my weekly chicken meal I could serve in many different appetising ways.

By now I felt that I had cleansed my body of all its ills and could therefore experiment further. My heavily filled teeth had for many years been prone to aches and twinges, particularly in cold weather, but since changing my diet the nerves in my teeth were much improved and I rarely had trouble with my teeth. This was a totally unexpected advantage that my new diet gave me.

I was always searching for a higher quality of life and to me this meant constantly improving my diet. I continued to listen to my body and to keep in tune with it always endeavouring for more harmony and balance. It was all so rewarding and by now the discipline of correct diet came completely naturally so that I never made the mistake of miscombining and so many pieces of my jigsaw were fitting into place more easily the more I learned. Now that I was feeling well it was all so much fun. I could experiment and if it didn't work out then I just tightened up on my original diet until my mistake was corrected and tried something else. Never be afraid to try out new ideas. They will be all your own, totally original, but the prize of good health makes the challenge irresistible.

One day whilst out I passed a group of children hungrily eating fish and chips with dirty greasy fingers from their packets wrapped in newspaper and this made me stop and think. Fish – why not try fish, not the chip shop variety but fresh fish, but all the wet fish shops that I knew of with their tiled and cold slabbed display counters seemed to have disappeared. This seemed dreadful as living on an island surrounded by seas which contained a variety of fish meant that we should grasp this underrated food which is high in protein and contains essential minerals and vitamins. Vitamins A, D and B group are the most important vitamins that fish contain together with the minerals calcium and iodine. They carry out a protective role in our bodies, ensuring that all the processes that had to occur to keep us alive and healthy happened smoothly and efficiently.

Different types of fish contained different amounts of fat. White fish like cod could contain as little as 1-2 per cent fat whilst oily fish like herring or trout vary from 10-20 per cent. Fish also contains a proportion of polyunsaturated fat which contributes to a healthier diet.

I seemed to remember long ago enjoying fresh plaice that I had watched my mother cook in the frying pan coating the freshly washed fillets in breadcrumbs and I would stand whilst the fish gently cooked and was placed on my plate with soft chips cooked in animal fat which gave a rich flavour. This was not the way for me any more but the memory of a long ago childhood edible pleasure was momentarily rekindled. Finding a small family run old fashioned wet fish shop just outside our town I called one morning surprised to find a queue of customers far outside the small shop door. Whilst waiting I viewed the fish on offer. There did not seem a great choice but what there was looked fresh and clean. Most of the customers seemed elderly and I watched each walk away after purchasing their choice wrapped in newspaper until it was my turn. I selected a small sized plaice which I had filleted and returned home. This I put into my steamer and paused – what would go with fish? Not chips! I didn't eat potatoes and besides that was bad combining. It had to be a vegetable as the fish would be the protein part of my meal. I surveyed the wealth of food in my refrigerator and instinctively knew that I would not put carrots with fish. I felt that it had to be a green vegetable. I alighted on a savoy cabbage and knew that this would make a harmonious meal. It was with much interest that I cooked this meal – together in my steamer – and watched as the fish turned white as it cooked and gave off an aroma that was new to me. This was the first time that I had ever steamed fish and I could hardly wait to sample my new meal. This I duly did with much pleasure, savouring each tender tasty mouthful until it was all eaten. I waited for the results. This meal was only slightly heavier than a nut or seed meal and certainly not as heavy as my chicken meal. I felt fine. There were no adverse reactions so I tried it again the following week with the same pleasure. After this I tried two generous cod cutlets which were much more meaty than the plaice but equally enjoyable with the savoy cabbage. As it was winter time there was not a great variety of green vegetables but as I enjoyed savoy so much this was most acceptable.

Steamed fish was now to become part of my diet, always eaten once a week but never more than twice. I shall always feel that any animal food should not be overindulged in and if in any doubt I would always give it a miss.

I only ever ate fish with one vegetable, usually green. This was a most attractive dish and perfectly satisfying . I was now so used to semi-mono meals that this was the way I prepared my meals and besides – I now much preferred this. The fewer food types in each meal the easier it was to savour the flavours and the more varied it made each meal.

All fish I enjoyed with spring as well as savoy cabbage and also broad beans and runner beans when in season. The more delicate flavoured vegetables were preferable so that the individuality of each fish was enhanced by its partner and not submerged. I now had this endless variety of fish to choose from and a whole new exciting sphere of eating had opened up for me. It was so long since I had eaten fish that it was all new to me and my next choice for trial was sole. Dover and lemon were the main two varieties. Both being flat the lemon sole was broader and smoother than the Dover. Lemon has a softer textured flesh but Dover has a slightly more positive flavour. These looked and always seemed to me easy to consume and an attractive addition to my culinary wardrobe.

Halibut was not always on display but instantly recognisable with its creamy colour and ridged flesh. Its firm texture with distinctive flavour cooperates well with steaming which always ensures that every particle of flavour is retained and helps keep the fish in a firm piece.

Of the white fish my first favourite has to be hake. A long silvery green fish with a firm flesh which tastes like no other, it is the one of which I never tire. Its body is small and strong and is at its most attractive when cut and steamed in steaks and eaten like all the other fish with a green vegetable. I consider silver hake my best friend of the undersea world.

Huss I eat occasionally as even with my fish meals I like as much variety as possible. This is long and round with a firm pink tinted flesh and mild in taste and I find not always available.

Whiting was one of the varieties of fish that I ventured to eat after seeing it many times but discarding it for a favourite. I should not have done this. It is a delightful fish and in appearance to me always seemed neat and tidy – being small and not as soft in texture as plaice and not as heavy as cod but definitely original in flavour and a whole small fish makes a satisfying meal. As it is comparatively free of bones there is no need to dissect the fish before eating.

Megrim when filleted can be mistaken for plaice but its skin is a pebbled grey with no orange spots. It is firmer than plaice and less sweet but a real delicacy. For a really different looking meal it is superb with shredded red cabbage, which when cooked changes colour to the deepest most royal purple.

It was with disappointment and concern that I learned that

the fish shop that I now frequented regularly was to close. I relied on that shop so much for such an important part of my diet I could not contemplate my life functioning without it. The owners now knew me well and would always recommend what to purchase from my repertoire.

After making extensive enquiries I was recommended to another small fish monger and it was most reluctantly that I made my first visit. There seemed quite a large variety of fish on sale and by now I considered myself quite an expert on the quality of fish and knew instinctively the good cuts to purchase that were on display.

I played safe and purchased some plaice fillets which I enjoyed. The following week I did the same with cod and gradually over the weeks became accustomed to another shop. Keith was the personable young man who now assisted me with my purchases and encouraged me to be more venturesome. For a while I was content to eat my usual favourites and he soon realised that if he had any hake for sale this is what I would purchase. I was amused when he told me I was referred to as "the hake lady".

One day Keith drew my attention to a large fish with a pink interior and silvery coat. He said it was wild river salmon and a real treat that he thought I should try as he had noticed that I never ate any oily fish. Over the months I had learned that his advice was invariably good and he cut me some thick steaks from the king of the freshwater fish.

The aroma as it cooked permeated my kitchen and the flesh darkened as it was ready to serve. Its texture was so different from anything that I had ever tasted and the flavour nothing short of edible ecstacy. From this day salmon was to be a real highlight of "fish days".

Another oily fish that Keith recommended that I try was trout. With a long speckled glossy solid little body, to be gutted then cooked and eaten in its entirety. As it cooked it resembled the salmon with its pink flesh but in flavour it was very much trout and superb to eat.

By now I had an infinite variety of sea food to enjoy and the pleasure of never knowing what would be on display on the different days. I also felt that fish caught naturally must surely be more free of contamination than the meat taken from sad miserable beasts forced to live their unhappy existences until slaughter was their only escape.

Whilst on holiday in Wales I visited a fish farm. Built only to help the existing fish, this ensured their existence. The trout were instantly recognisable with their specked bodies and I was happy to see them swimming rather than on the cold slab which was more familiar to me. I felt anything that could help nature was good and I was surprised to learn that a number of years passed before the fish – being transferred from one tank to another as they grew – were large enough to be released which did seem most fitting for this graceful creature. I was fascinated to see the fish lift designed to help fish overcome the weir and the fish ladder to help them climb the falls. I find it gratifying amidst modern technology and sophisticated equipment that such time and patience had been given to help not only assisting the trout to survive but actually contributing to giving them a better quality of life and also allowing people to learn and appreciate their life cycle in their river home beneath the rolling mountains.

My body always seemed happy and better for my fish meals and these are now part of my eating for health lifestyle. As with all my other food I buy as fresh as possible and keep in the refrigerator until ready to cook, after being washed thoroughly first in running cold water. Another benefit is that fish freezes perfectly so I am always able to buy a little extra of my particular favourites and keep it for the times when I am unable to visit the shop. Of course the best of having fish in my diet is that it tastes so delicious and is therefore a joy to consume.

Over the months since I had introduced animal protein into my diet I did feel generally much stronger and had more stamina and felt that I needed some meat and fish in my diet, but never more than one chicken and at most two fish meals a week.

I considered that I had achieved remarkable results and was now unrecognisable from the more dead than alive pitiful being of all those months ago. Although I had adapted easily and contentedly to my new diet and now felt it was as good as I was able to have it, I thought of my favourite foods that I had given up in my get-well quest and as I had had no adverse symptoms with the introduction of animal protein I decided to experiment a little further. One of my favourite foods was Cheddar cheese and this had now been absent from my diet from its initial change to healthy eating. Of course it could not be with a rich brown crusty piece of bread which was my usual way as this was a combination not to be accepted by a conscious combiner at any price. I decided to try it out as a main meal with lightly cooked cauliflower florets. I didn't cook the cheese and I now decided only to use the vegetarian variety that was not made with animal rennet. I sliced it into pieces and with a small amount of sea salt ate it with my crunchy cauliflower. I tasted each delicious mouthful with the added delight of knowing that this meal was well out-of-bounds and afterwards waited anxiously for my body to protest. It didn't! I was delighted. I tried it the following week. I had the same enjoyment of such a simple but tasty meal prepared and cooked in the minimum amount of time. Like all animal derived meals it was slightly heavier than the nut and seed ones but as I did not consume a large amount of cheese I found that my body was quite happy with this. I was convinced now that as I was so improved in health I could consume an added forbidden delight as eating a much loved food certainly gave me a great mind lift.

For my mid-afternoon drink I now sometimes had Luaka decaffeinated tea. This delectable beverage is most refreshing and one cup a day is always a welcome treat. Coffee I never miss but admit to finding its aroma quite intoxicating.

During the evenings when I was relaxing with my family Brian liked chocolate and toffees but would always suck them slowly whilst Jamie would chew his in seconds. I felt that I would like a snack before bedtime. Sometimes I would have a dish of gorgeous porridge made of Mornflake organic oats and my favourite Volvic mineral water, topped if I felt the desire for something sweet with a spoonful of Applefords black strap molasses. I had also treated myself to some biscuits made without animal fat from the health shop. These made a sustaining snack without being too heavy for an evening meal. Sometimes I would have thin rounds of granary bread crisply toasted and topped with butter, but usually I had porridge and biscuits or porridge and large round rice biscuits. I rarely felt the need for the sweetness of the nutritious carob bars.

Once the body is accustomed to an ideal diet you will never crave for the wrong foods or wish to overindulge in anything. Enjoyment will be paramount and the body naturally regulates the amount it requires. Teach your body to know what is beneficial to it. It will be an apt pupil and learn quickly and will soon let you know if you put something inside it that offends in any way. It wants help and will soon discipline itself to accept the correct amounts of wholesome foods. Let your body enjoy its power and let it help you achieve perfect health. Your body has a vested interest in getting well. Be friends with it and live in perfect accord. Joy and harmony will be your reward.

Like most people I did my bulk shopping only once a week and I soon found that my fridge door just would not shut with a mountain of lettuce and green vegetables plus everything else that I needed. I had not envisaged re-designing my rather antiquated kitchen but I soon realised that I would have to do exactly this. A large base unit full of now unnecessary utensils was discarded and in its place installed a new larder fridge. Likewise my freezer was unable to hold all the summer goodies that were so necessary for the following twelve months of fresh organic raspberries, blackberries and runner beans as well as bulky granary loaves. In came two new freezers and I was thankful not to have a weekly juggle to fit everything in. Two fridges and three freezers may sound a lot but believe me I could easily use more. However I manage and live on fresh or frozen fresh food and would not have it otherwise. Give yourself plenty of good storage space and you will be rewarded by a daily supply of appetising health-giving food sitting patiently in your own kitchen shop just waiting to be eaten.

Another fascinating discovery was that not only did I now automatically combine the correct foods for each meal, my body would now tell me the way it wanted me to plan the whole days eating menu. All my meals were perfectly acceptable to me whilst being consumed in perfect rotation, but my body would tell me that it preferred a certain fruit breakfast with a particular type of lunch following. For example, grapes were an ideal light breakfast if lunch was to be a heavy meal of, say, cheese or chicken. A more solid breakfast of apple combined with a berry fruit was fine when followed by a lighter type lunch of green vegetables and a light nut like almonds. I also found that after a cheese and cauliflower meal containing no greens for my evening salad my body preferred plenty of lettuce with either cress or watercress. These revelations were fascinating and I was finding that to give my body exactly what it wanted was the sure road to complete health. To be in such total harmony with my body and having now such highly developed sensitivity to all its needs was exhilarating in the extreme.

As my new wonder diet gave me back my good health and helped restore all the lost energy, I was eager to enter into the world and really live again in the way that I had been unable to do now for so long. I had no intention of foregoing my diet and there was no need to do this on our outings when it was so easy to pack up an appetising salad meal for a picnic to be shared during our explorations of the countryside and river banks.

Holidays away from home I was determined to participate in to the full and do now as a normal years holidays have five separate weeks staggered throughout the school holiday year. For many years we have opted out of the hotel type holidays as fixed meal times were taboo when on holiday and we gained much pleasure on sending for and browsing through mountains of holiday literature before deciding on the best holiday apartments that we could find. If it was to be a seaside holiday then the flat had to overlook the sea and if inland it just must have a fine view, plenty of space and as much comfort as was available. This guaranteed a relaxing time away from the pressures of everyday life and was a great enhancer to fitness. By trial and error I found I much preferred still to prepare my own food as I now had an inbred suspicion of most prepared foods. When we did eat out I much preferred the largest busiest establishment that could be found as this usually would give the most extensive menu where I could normally find something suitable and if well frequented then I assumed that the turnover in food would be brisk and therefore the food would be reasonably fresh. All cooked meals I immediately found seemed well over-cooked by my standards and therefore nutritionally under par and I found the popular carvery where you could choose your own food the best suited to my requirements. If I found just everything unpalatable then I could always have a handful of nuts or seeds and to date have managed quite well as our days outings always included a salad meal that I would consume with even more eagerness than usual if the previous meal had been a scratch affair.

Eating out in company even at a set meal can usually be coped with without having to offend your palate. Just remember to combine correctly and if in doubt leave. Never be without your own little back-up goody bag as you will surprisingly find that the most elevated establishments can only do conventional meals and if the main course is a badly combined dish like meat or fish pie then you will have problems unless you choose to dissect the pie. Personally I find it easier to discard such miscombinations and settle for the freshest least cooked vegetables that are offered. If you are invited to a meal at a friends house where the numbers are likely to be few and the hostess to have spent hours concocting her most memorable masterpiece then this can be difficult, but as you have no wish to lose a friend or change your way of eating then you must speak to your hostess well prior to the meal and explain your diet. If she is a close friend she will probably know of it already and make sure that there is something that you can enjoy. If not, tell her quite truthfully that you will be happy to provide your own food and besides, it is her company that you want most anyway. Explain that to you your diet is as important as medication is to most people and in no way would anyone stop someone taking their medication. This should work and if not, well then, you have a choice of the friend or the diet. My friends now are those who understand me and accept me as I am. They are usually mystified by my determination but intrigued that it means so much to me and that I like it so well. It is an ingrained part of me not ever to be deviated from. This just happens to be my way of coping and remember, if you cheat too much then you won't be on a diet at all and there is no way you want to go on the downhill spiral is there? My diet was sacrosanct, but in no way parochial as I would always welcome improvement and as a perquisite of a perfect diet I knew that I would never again be emaciated

In *Man The Unknown*, nobel prize-winner Dr. Alexis Carrel made two profound observations; 'There is no doubt that consciousness is affected by the quantity and quality of the food... The Possession of natural health would enormously increase the happiness of man.' This surely proves that the Hay system offers an important and wholly beneficial dimension not only for avoiding degenerative disease, but for successful, healthy and happy living.

This diet is so varied and life-giving I wonder now how I ever survived without it. By choice I shall never deviate from my chosen way of life as I know without any doubt that without a good diet good health cannot be regained. Actresses Caroline Blackiston, Lady Patience in Brass and Brenda

Bruce, Jenny Seagrove, Millicent Martin, Koo Stark and Cher are exponents of the Hay diet, also actor Sir John Gielgud and I have also read that the Duchess of York has been initiated to it.

My diet is no chore, it is the most delightful way of eating that I could ever envisage. Eat until satisfied of nutritious food correctly combined and any weight irregularity will restore its balance and this is why I can happily contemplate eating in this way forever.

Always I was making new discoveries. I had thought that finding the secret of healthy eating would be the end of my search for good health, but I was wrong. It was the most important aspect, but like climbing a mountain, you reach what you think is the top only to find more and more peaks. I still had more peaks to scale.

11

EXERCISE AND FRESH AIR

E xercise and fresh air are essential for good health and without them no-one can be completely well. All of my life I had enjoyed being outside in all weathers so this was something that I did not have to learn, just to make sure that I did it regularly and properly to gain optimum benefit from this natural medicine.

When young and totally fit strenuous exercise can be participated in with enjoyment and my simple pleasure as a child of roller skating around the quiet pavements where I lived with other local children was great fun. I did not have the modern roller skate boots of today but the metal variety that we strapped to our shoes and used until the wheels wore out and the metal ball bearing showed. As I became older I graduated to the far easier ice skates and liked the smell of the cold rinks with wet patches of ice to be avoided and can easily recall the sound of the clash of metal blades and the soft swish of perfect arcs cut in the ice and the dull thud of well executed landings from intricate jumps. Rounders was easily my favourite competitive game and playing for my school house was great fun and made for tremendous rivalry with healthy competition from friends in other houses. I was a force to be reckoned with as my house team bowler and enjoyed every minute of my success. Tennis was another sport that I participated in for many years and the vigorous set that I played daily with my friend Chris as we became keen to do well was tiring but rewarding as we sat, hot and dishevelled as we gulped refreshing water after our lunchtime sessions. Swimming – that most relaxing of all exercises – has been a lifetime's pleasure. It was not for me to do one powerful length after another, but lazily to become at one with the lift of the water, cutting it with slow strokes and breathing deeply and feeling the whole body benefit and the bliss of floating weightlessly. I can vividly recall the cacophony of sound at the local swimming baths as I gazed up at the ceiling and felt quite apart from the other swimmers as my body moved pleasurably in the cool water even in those early years. It was so different from being in the sea feeling the pull of a heavy swell and the tangy smell of the sea and suddenly being jolted into spluttering on becoming engulfed in an unnoticed wave cascading over my face and filling my nostrils with sea water.

As I grew older I derived much pleasure from long country walks with my father and the lessons in nature that he would give me, pointing out trees, drawing my attention to the different shapes and different colours of the leaves. There was the satisfaction of walking on natural surfaces of grass or soil or sand in preference to concrete and tarmac and of scrambling down the eerie Seven Sisters caverns on our local Wrens Nest; exercise for the mind and body of young inquisitive people. There was the harder exercise of climbing mountains in our beloved North Wales. Special climbs were shared with my father and Uncle Bob and Jan, like the still hot day in mid-summer when the four of us climbed the real mountain of Cader Idris, our climb starting in Arthog, past the lovely Llyn Crogenen and over the saddle and climbing steadily until we reached the summit. Jan and myself were twelve years old and in my youthful athleticism bounded to the top determined to be first to scale the 2927 feet. The achievement was a great one for us girls as we sat breathing heavily after our physical exertions, our bodies etched against an azure sky as we gazed at the vast expanse of God's beautiful creation in awed silence and then with longing at the lakes far below in want of a refreshing drink. Our descent was a scramble down the famous Foxes Path and then we welcomed the ice cold water of Llyn-y-Cafr to quench our parched throats. We walked to Dolgellau to catch the train home where excitedly we told our waiting mothers of our expedition.

Like most young people of my time I had a bicycle. Not one of the sophisticated models of today but the conventional old fashioned school girl variety that I and my contemporaries had. They were a necessity to arrive at school as I lived a considerable distance from any school and by today's standards the roads were quiet and we girls would ride together in convoys quite safe from vehicles and our bicycles would be left in rows of concrete blocks with no risk from vandals. I enjoyed riding around the countryside where I lived at the weekends, sometimes alone and sometimes with my best friend Rosemarie. We would puff inelegantly up the steep hills knowing that all the effort would be worth it for the exhilarating whizz down with the wind streaming our hair and cooling our hot faces. My bicycle was a treasured possession for many years.

Water I have always loved from the early days when I would play by the dark waters of the canals in Tipton running and jumping with youthful agility in places that I should not have been and enjoying the forbidden delight of crossing the canals by walking over the lock gates with the water high on one side and the deep drop into the still water far below me broken only by water oozing from the wooden gates making a dirty foam. I never fell in and still enjoy the serenity of hidden waterways giving a tranquil beauty, all the more poignant when found in our local industrial towns.

The sea I always hold in great respect having seen it in all its moods but nothing can match the pleasure and thrill of dinghy sailing in a fresh wind on an ever so slightly choppy sea. To hear the creak of wood, the pull of the wind in the sails and the reassuring steadying of the centreboard, to sit out so far that your hair trails in the water and view the wet world of wavelets lapping against a clinker-built hull from a new angle is a most satisfying experience equalled only by the feeling of planing, with the wind hard behind and lifting the dinghy so that the keel lightly kisses the water. It was exciting exercise and hard work and there was nothing quite like returning home covered in salt spray after being so close to nature that you were part of it.

Running is a perfect way to keep fit when you are young and I would often break into a run from sheer pleasure of having a healthy body full of energy, not sprinting or jogging but running lightly and in rhythmic movement until my whole body was aglow. Every part of it would be in unison and perfect accord.

These were my favourite forms of exercise through my life and they have given me much pleasure and satisfaction and I am glad that I participated in them all when I was young and able to enjoy them to the full. Now I am content to indulge in the more sedate exercise of walking, but it is no less beneficial and if done regularly and correctly will give the body all the movements that it needs to stay healthy. I try to walk twice daily, always first thing in the morning when joints need to be flexed after a nights sleep and also when the air is at its cleanest. There is nothing more welcoming than that first deep breath of fresh air as I walk outside for the first time. Whatever the weather is like makes no difference – it is fresh air and absolutely essential to good health. Always walk in comfortable flat shoes. Feet were not meant to be elevated into grotesque shapes. Always wear natural fibres in all clothes as far as is possible to enable the skin to breath. Cotton in summer and wool in winter are ideal. When walking keep to a pace that is comfortable, not a hurry nor a stroll but an evenly paced walk with good posture. Whenever possible walk on natural ground – a field or the sea shore. When inland walk on grass if possible. This is more natural for feet than a pavement or hard concrete. Your body will benefit from walking on natural ground, from summer sun to soft snow and squelchy wet fields. I love all the seasons. Keep the body relaxed with head erect and everything else will automatically be right. Imagine someone gently pulling the hair on top of your head straight up and this immediately takes pressure off all bones and assists joints to move easily. This is of great benefit to arthritic sufferers and my own bones have greatly improved in mobility since I have given my body correct balance and it will help you to walk tall and lightly on your feet. You will feel quite buoyant and concentrate on obtaining a good walking posture until it becomes second nature to you. Walks of a quarter of an hour twice daily are all that is needed to assist your body achieve fitness. It is far better to do two small walks, or even one, regularly than a days walk occasionally. This could strain your body if it is not used to it and the aim is to get fit in the most pleasing way possible so that it becomes such a pleasure that the exercise will be participated in with eagerness. Many people include a daily walk into their busy routine and never deviate from it wherever they are. Ayatollah Khomeini was one; in his old age he would walk daily for twenty minutes and if returning before this time had passed he would go back even for an extra few minutes.I am sure this gentle but regular routine assisted him to live to old age. Yasser Arafat is another; in his dangerous and busy world his exercise is compulsive. He always walks briskly each day for thirty minutes regardless of where he is and whatever commitments he has. Even when confined for safety he always fits in his walk. I understand how these people feel. Walking not only sets the body into correct motion for the day but gives the mind a lift too. Regular walking helps the whole body fit into place and is as necessary as eating good food. The body muscles become weak with lack of proper exercise and if not used for a period of ten days lose a third of their strength.

The special plus of walking is that anyone can do it and fit the distance walked and the speed to individual needs and although I sometimes think of more strenuous exercise, I know that my daily walk is essential to my well-being.

As air is essential to live it is obvious that the best quality air obtainable should be used. To walk through busy towns and along congested roads is not the time for deep relaxing breathing but the benefit is immediately enhanced in your own rear garden or in the centre of a park even if it is near to a town. I am fortunate in having a rear garden that backs on to the natural grounds of the local Zoo and which is free from contamination and a haven for wild life. I also have natural parklands for my daily walks which I utilise to the full. The important thing is to make the best of the facilities available. If you do live in a busy area then early in the morning when the air is freshest is the best time for exercising your body and filling it with the purest air that is so vital. It never ceases to amaze me that all the things best for us are natural and free. Of course the best air is obtained outside but this does not mean that your home should be neglected. In summer most people have windows open but in winter all are firmly closed to retain central heating warmth.

My windows are open all year round and these should be as clean as possible to allow the maximum amount of light in when they are closed. I will leave a bedroom window open in a heatwave during the night which is something that I normally never do. Net curtains should be avoided wherever possible as they obscure light, in daytime curtains should be drawn well off windows. I have never personally found the night air beneficial but counteract that by opening the bedroom window on rising and only closing up when retiring. All the windows in the house are similarly open and I much prefer to put on an extra layer of clothing than have a fire on. Having been brought up all my life in a house with no central heating I don't find it necessary and even in my sitting room I find a gas fire put on an hour before the room is used will warm it adequately even in the coldest weather. I find a gas fire preferable to an electric one and an open fire preferable to both. Nostalgia takes me back to my childhood when every home had an open fire which gave a welcoming warmth in the depths of winter and a comforting cosiness as it died away during late evening, where sitting in the firelight conjuring pictures in the red embers of spent coal and logs made a magic natural world of a healthy heat that the majority of today's children have never even seen.Then there was the task of raking the still warm ashes the following morning and sorting the cinders to be used for the next fire from the bats to be discarded and laying the small pieces of wood and twisted newspapers and placing the small pieces of coal with the cinders as the small flames licked the paper into charred slivers. A gentle blow from my mother was all that was needed to ensure a success, not like my early efforts of energetic blowing that left me with no fire but a black face. It was so satisfying to see the flames spurt up the chimney with of course the occasional excitement of the chimney catching fire. I remember this happening to us and sitting tense as the soot caught fire and the flames roared in the chimney and the chimney breast was hot to the touch. It was all part of a departed way of life that was more healthy and natural.

I have always liked a cool atmosphere in the home and my family often say that germs could not survive in such a temperature. As we rarely have seasonal ailments of coughs and colds and in five years at school Jamie has only had one day off due to illness I feel that my lifestyle is successful for all of us. I feel positively miserable in the normal overheated home with its suffocating atmosphere due to retaining all heat. It invariably gives me a headache and if accompanied by cigarette smoke I find it purgatory.

Recently while journeying in a heavily laden car to our holiday destination on the south coast our car completely failed at the southern end of the M1 motorway which was some considerable distance from home. After the expert opinion of the motorway maintenance mechanic and calling out a breakdown service man both informed us that the car could not be repaired and we would have to be towed ignominiously home. It was suggested by the service engineer that I travel in his van as guide and Brian steer our car while being towed and Jamie stay with him. I said I preferred us to travel together when he apologetically informed us that we would not be able to use the car heater. After the strain of the breakdown this caused us instant relaxation as we burst into laughter. The poor man had no idea what he had said to cause such merriment until Brian informed him that we never used the heater and invariably travelled with a window open in all weathers. I recoiled in horror at his comfortable warm van and travelled on tow with Brian and Jamie until the last few miles when I was needed as a guide. I could hardly concentrate on the directions as my nose became stuffy and my eyes smarted and it was with much relief in many ways when we returned home. The A A mechanic was happy but sympathetic and the service he provided was of the highest calibre. We shall always be grateful to their relay service coming to our aid within minutes of our distress call but I am sure he wondered what sort of people he had been called out to save.

To complement the fresh air in the house I like a variety of green plants. Not only does having living things give an interest as they grow but they are beneficial to the air and green is the most restful of colours. Green is the colour of peace and a living green plant in all the downstairs rooms of the house gives an immediate aura of serenity. They do not exude any scent but an enveloping calmness, particularly if sitting adjacent to them. To watch plants grow is to have a portion of nature in your home and patiently watching its evolution will bring you peace and fulfilment. I was interested to learn that Spider plants are thought to be good at "eating" pollutants such as benzene, carbon monoxide and formaldehyde. I never have cut flowers with their heady perfumes that offend my nostrils – besides from my animal rights days I felt it unkind to cut a flower in its prime when it should be left to enjoy the fresh air and sunlight as it was meant to.

My family have lived in our present home for over ten years and like most people we wanted this to be full of our own personal items and decorated to our choice. As daylight and lightness are essential to wellbeing any paintwork that was redecorated was done in white. Walls were papered in light colours and as carpets were replaced these were also in light colours. Many people said how unwise this was with a young boisterous son causing many muddy footprints as he and his friends went in and out. I disagreed and chose the best wool quality available in multi-colours but predominately white or cream and they keep surprisingly clean and, most important, give an immediate air of lightness which is uplifting. Being of natural fibres it is also beneficial to walk on with bare feet – likewise wooden floors. These are ideal to walk on as they are full of strength which will enter the body so it is good to have as many of natures blessings in your home as possible. The inside of a house should copy the outside and be full of health-giving light. There should be nothing heavy and overpowering as this gives the mind a downward spiral whereas lightness and airiness give immediate mental and physical uplift. Never have heavy light shades and only use artificial lights when absolutely necessary. Natural light is good for health and as the day ends and it becomes darker eyes adjust accordingly and will not feel tired if used without any artificial aid even in dusk. What is more relaxing than sitting in a room in an evening with the only light from a fire. Artificial light when needed should only be gentle, never anything harsh that will give glare and hurt eyes. Keep your home and life as light as possible and this will give you bodily and mental uplift.

Many people think that only sunlight is good for the body but this is not so. Remember that natural daylight is also important. On the dullest most miserable day the light will be far better than the harsh artificial lights emitted from most houses. The body needs to be outside to absorb whatever light can be obtained from every day. Be greedy about natural light and allow your body the opportunity to soak up as much as is possible. This is most important in seeking good health.

Daily exercise is necessary all year round but of course it is most enjoyable in the warmth of summer sunshine. Sitting in the sunlight in the morning before the heat becomes too intense and late afternoon or early evening is advantageous, not only in giving the body vitamin D, but in toning the skin and being, I find, the most pleasing form of relaxation. Two sessions daily with eyes closed is also good for eyes. Never use a sun cream. If the sun is too hot don't sit in it. I never use sun creams and never burn as I listen to my body as it always tells me when to sit in the sunshine and for how long. Always give your body plenty of unstrained exercise and fresh air with sunshine when available and you will have learned another important part of my health-giving lifestyle.

12

NATURE

An affinity with nature is an essential part of my lifestyle and with daily walks in the fresh air who can be unaware of the beauty around us. An appreciation of the seasons of the year brings a wealth o f beauty and wonder.

Who cannot quicken with the coming of spring and the start of a new year. To be in accord with nature helps the body and mind to develop and grow just as the seasons grow. Buds appear bravely to challenge the end of winter as they bring a pale green to the barren trees and open in shining newness as spring arrives. There are the first snowdrops in a country lane and the lesser celandine with its goldenstar-like petals that are unmistakable and if you search you can find the small wild daffodils buffeted in the spring gales. Violets hide under protecting trees which soar with outstretched branches reaching for the sky from the solid reassuring earth from which all goodness grows. The pale sky has clouds tattered by a March wind light as gossamer as they are tossed at random.

It is not necessary to be a nature expert to appreciate it. The might of an oak tree is sturdy and reliable and oh so English. The Copper Beech has rich deep coloured leaves unfurling now that spring has come and the dainty graceful birch shows its silver bark. There is the proud upright poplar and the rounded horse chestnut. All have their appeal in such differing shapes and colours.

Trees would not be complete without a mention of the birds who live in them and find safety in their cover. Birds are so much more than varieties of feathers enhancing the sky. They all have their special differences not only as species but as individuals. As you become familiar with birds you appreciate that some are much more timid than others and some venturesome and listen when you talk to them. Some come in pairs, others in groups and of course there are loners. Their calls are so different. Some hop on the ground with jerky jumps and others take sedate steps while birds so elegant in the air can appear cumbersome on the ground.

Enjoy the regular birds in your area and look forward with interest at seeing different species when visiting new parts of the country. Watching and learning about birds can be fascinating and making friends with your own special ones gives a keen sense of satisfaction if you have the patience to let these tiny treasures of the sky know that you are no foe. The house sparrow looks small and defenceless but is well able to look after itself. The pied wagtail, smart in its mourning colours hops jerkily in search of worms and does not mind me gazing at him as he enjoys his meal. Notice the sleek blackbird with melodious voice and polite speckled thrush. The immaculately groomed magpies always seem to be in pairs. I have a number of regular pairs visit and they look after each other well but are not so kind to their fellow birds, and their raucous chatter is instantly recognisable. The bright chirpy robin is associated with the chill of winter but I have a friend who visits all the year round and is now tame enough to hop beside me on the wheelbarrow and watch me at my garden toils. The male pheasant can often be seen in the countryside a blaze of colour with its proud plumage.

Shropshire Spring lambs are unsteady ontheir feet and always remind me of Siamese cats with their black faces, ears and legs. They are more sturdy than the similarly coloured Suffolk sheep and so different from the long faced small Welsh mountain sheep that flourish on the scrubby Welsh hillsides. The Kent sheep with heavy fleece of long crimpy wool are always to be seen on Romney Marsh so aptly called green and white by Malcolm Saville.

Late spring when it is good to be in the clean air of the country shows the bluebell giving the earth a misty purple haze against the bark of the trees which is complemented by their deep green leaves and white stems. Never pick them, they should be left to adorn the ground as nature intended. All wild flowers wilt in sadness when they are picked and are only happy when admired and left to adorn another country day.

In summer when nature is fully matured and magical in its beauty and all trees clothed in dense green foliage noisily alive with bird life, thoughts of people living in towns dwell on visits to the seaside where another world is waiting to be explored. The wet sand that oozes soggily through toes when walking along the edge of the sea gradually becomes hot to the touch as you move away from the sea into the soft sand with pebbles burning bare toes. Fine trickling sand amidst dunes with their spiky strands sigh in a gentle breeze, never more prolific than in Abersoch. It is a haven for contented crickets in the heat of midsummer where all is sea and sky and sand, unpolluted by sounds other than those of welcome nature. Walking lightly over a pebbly beach under cliffs one gazes up at sandmartins busily making their fragile homes.

The herring gulls at Llandudno and the yellow broom in the sands of Southwold are two contrasting vivid seaside memories. The sandy terrain near the sea has its own colours of the varying pinks of sturdy thrift, clinging to wind-battered cliffs with determined tenacity at Trefor on the Llyn Penisula and at New Quay in Mid Wales. Who hasn't enjoyed searching for shells as a child and it is just as enjoyable a pastime for an adult. Scratching for the secrets of the sand on Mochras in North Wales surrounded by silver gilt sea and the endless cry of seabirds can make time stand still with natures music broken only by exclamations of delight as a special shell is discovered. The common top shell can be whitest white or a pearly hue. The spiral of the common wentle trap and tower shells vary from the common limpet. The small strong ridged arctic cowrie so different from the evenly shaped razor shell which is so brittle and the pearly pink common tellin peep up from their hiding place in the sand. Queen scallop of pink and white and the variegated scallop when collected, brought home and washed and glued to plant pots to make an individual memento will evoke a memory of a summer day.

Over the years I have found pleasure in exploring rock pools and there is an abundance of these in Criccieth, some quite shallow in water warm to an enquiring foot and some surprisingly deep and cold. These pools support plants and creatures which cannot survive in more exposed places and by repeated visits to the same pool you can recognise the resident inhabitants from the visitors who come and go with each tide. An empty pool at first glance can be seen to be full of living things on closer inspection. On the beach at Criccieth numerous crabs can be found of varying sizes and tenacity together with gently waving anemonies and rocks slippery with green seaweed. Brown seaweed is also to be found on the pebble beach with its all-engulfing health-giving smell. I bring some home and place it on the garden and on walking past it take in deep breaths, filling my lungs with its unique aroma, closing my eyes and being a hundred miles away at my favourite seaside. The pebbles on this beach are unsurpassable and in unbelievable colours and shapes, hardly seeming natural and I have many specimens to remind me of them. It is so noisy when the sea recedes from them and pulls them into the sea on a squally day and so quiet with a mild sea lapping over them on a calm day.

Before leaving the beach feel the sun warming your body with a penetration to make your bones feel pliant, breathe the clean air and gaze at the beauty around you. Walk along and love every minute of it and if you feel like it run for sheer pleasure at the happiness being part of such a scene can bring.

Picnicking in the peace of Ynys-y-Pandy with the trickling stream the only sound to break the stillness and the occasional plop of a fish coming to the surface we sit in the shade of the mill, its gaunt ruins standing proud against the azure sky. Searching the banks I explore for flowers and find the palest blue field scabious and on an open patch of dry soil the little red tinted yellow blooms of the birdsfoot trefoil with its intricate shape, growing in clusters close to the ground. Its curious name seems to have come about because the flowers are followed by little seedpods which, when clustered together, look rather like a birds claw. The neat little plant spreads rapidly under taller grasses and can sometimes change the appearance of a field or a dry bank giving a rich royal gold and maroon carpet of soft brightness. Walk upstream with only dragonflies for company where trees heavy in their summer coats of green give shade and explore until you can find wild blackberries fully ripe with an invitation to be eaten. They stain your fingers black as the juice oozes onto them and one becomes aware of the familiar woody smell as one puts one's face near the inky blackness.

My gaze alights on a dark brown object moving with speed along the grass. It is a furry caterpillar infrequently seen now but a reminder to me of long ago summers when all gardens held an abundance of these delights of summer. We children would carefully collect them and place them in jam jars before transferring them to a grand home made of discarded shoe boxes with an outdoor run made of our mother's nylons attached to twigs. I would wait until evening and look at my captives. Most curled and still and being troubled by their captivity I would gently tip them out onto the grass. I would be content to watch them busily going about their business free as they should be. They did not mind as I lightly ran my small enquiring finger along their soft fur. They knew me for a friend.

It seems a paradox that I relish being encompassed in the smell of freshly cut grass and hay and the peaty aroma of sodden earth and the delicate scent of heather covering Welsh mountains and the rich ripe joy of wild blackberries and strawberries, yet bottled perfumes of flower imitations clog my nose and bring tears to my eyes and give me an immediate headache. I have often wondered why the strong smell of tar that was so frequently spread on the road when I was a child gave me such an uplift when taking deep breaths of its pungent smell, until I realised that it was not a man-made substance at all but a black viscous by-product from the distillation of coal. I would follow the lumbering steam roller as it rumbled along getting its treacle ware over myself and my clothes but unable to leave its intoxicating smell. In later years I was to learn from my father-in-law who worked for a tar distillery that tar was most beneficial to chests and that no-one who worked at the distillery ever suffered with catarrh. Venturing further I find a hidden lake with silken sheen in the heat of summer stillness, surrounded by rolling mountains lazily changing contour as the shade of a passing cloud gives a darker hue to the gentle green.

The largest and most common of the British wild roses is the dog-rose which can, like the honeysuckle, be found in the hedgerow. In spite of what I feel is an inappropriate name, for the flowers are fragrant with large heart-shaped petals of pink and white, the fruits of the wild rose are the scarlet berries from which rose-hip syrup is made. The hips can be seen thick in the hedge in the autumn. For me the wild rose and the honeysuckle with its unmistakable heady sweet smell and yellow red tinged flowers rich in nectar frequented by bees and moths seem partners as even with flowers so different both have sweet smells and berries to brighten the end of summer and are tough-stemmed and able to survive their hedgerow rivals. Honeysuckle is also visited by butterflies of unimaginable exquisiteness. The large and small tortoise-shell, rusty red with jagged wing tips and mighty red admiral of dramatic red and black and white come to mind. The large and small white really looks more lemon than white with dark dusty markings and bright yellow brimstone, happy in its summer colour. The dainty small common blue is found in sighing grasslands and so many more, living out their short lives in a miriad of colours to add to the wonder of nature. The

Buddlia imported from the Far East in 1890 and known as the butterfly tree due to these beauties of summer being attracted to the perfume of the long mauve flowers should be encouraged. Have one in your garden and you will reap the reward of many varieties of butterfly visitors.

Daintiest of all the wild flowers must surely be the frail looking harebell, its exquisite blue bell hanging suspended as a water droplet from the slimmest of stems as it brightens a grassy bank. Gently tip up the bell and look at its misty interior and it is easy to imagine the gentle tinkling it would make as the slightest kiss of wind will cause it to swing in graceful curves.

If you are lucky you can find wild strawberries, with dainty flowers before bursting into the deepest pink fruit that is a joy to find and pick and eat.

All of natures gifts enrich life and it is all there for everyone to search for its treasure trove.

Explore the mountains high above Blaenau Ffestiniog and wonder at the scene far below while picking wild dark bilberries and of course the blackberries of North Wales are larger, blacker and more succulent than anywhere.

The rhythmic call of a cuckoo on a summer day can be heard while sitting high on the Berwyns engulfed in sweet scented heather of every hue of pink and mauve. Walk along the rough sheep tracks where sheep are the only companions for us as we visit favourite secret haunts far away from civilisation.

Swans – many of them – familiar and unafraid gracefully gild the waters of Porthmadog Harbour as they glide regally by. The small chunky mallards and tufted ducks to be found on lazy summer rivers are always in abundance on the river Severn at Stourport where they give immense pleasure to the passengers of the craft on the river.

Summer is my favourite time with all its fullness of beauty and warmth that invades the body and soul but all too soon the golden fields of corn appear interspersed with a partially hidden dot of red as a poppy can be seen when the ripe stems are moved like a gentle sea and the wind makes itself felt. Soon all will be cut and harvested and early autumn will come bringing the most colourful of the seasons where all is golden and mellow. Trees in their majesty are holders of secrets of history as their years pass and they reach maturity. The trees cling vainly to those once green leaves now turning delicately gold and as they turn to rust falling hesitantly to the ground as if suspended on silken threads on a magical Indian summer day when the air is so still that you can hear the quiet, the sun still giving mellow warmth as it casts ever lengthening shadows across the carpet of golden leaves. These are days to visit the country and pick the last blackberries of the season in the warmth of protected bushes and ponder with satisfaction on a year now half over.

The woodmouse who is so tame he will keep himself busy outside my back door during summer and is often in danger of being squashed as he basks in the sun is not so often seen with the chill nip in the air that can now be felt in the late afternoon. Wood pigeons, the fattest I have ever seen who waddled with ungain gait on my lawn and onto the rocks of my pond all summer have gone away now to find a safe haven for winter but will return again next spring.

The grey squirrels in paradise in the woods near to me eagerly pick up the acorns that I collect for them and busily bury so many that I should be surrounded by a forest of oak trees. They are so agile and quick, having no fear of me when I scold them for eating my strawberries and stealing my apples.

Hedgehogs hide in the now fast growing pile of golden bronze leaves and are content to be carried to a safer place and I have an old dog kennel for their use. It is a fallacy that they like bread and milk. No adult animal of any species drinks milk, they obtain it from their mother's when they are babies but scraps of meat or dog food with a shallow dish of clean water will be gratefully partaken by any nocturnal visitors.

The fox family that has graced our garden with their presence for many years and is now sufficiently tame to stay in the garden at the same time as I am outside is a delight to watch. Young cubs will come up to the kitchen window and look up at me while a parent watches from a distance. Apart from a few holes in the lawn these beautiful animals cause none of the damage so often unfairly attributed to them and with the coming of autumn their magnificent coats perfectly blend with the golden world now evolving. They have dug themselves a hole under my fence and come for the regular food I give them. They like chicken and any kind of meat soon disappears and the interest and satisfaction in watching these animals live out their natural lives as they should is infinitely rewarding and I am glad that they choose me as a human they can trust. Never forget that these wild animals should never be encouraged as house pets but appreciated in their natural habitat and just by observing it is possible to learn so much about them.

All the rabbits abundant in the summer moorland now disappear for warmth in their homes as the days shorten. The sky with its endless variety of apparel is now blemished with the gathering dark clouds scudding in the first heavy wind slanting the rain fiercely onto the trees causing the valiantly clinging leaves to fall in golden showers onto the ground in waves of sodden wet colour. As the days pass the branches become more apparent as a freak storm curves mighty trees into a chorus of quarter moons as the last leaves are torn off to a form of thick carpet of burnished gold to scuffle through, all bronze and deepest plum shades and some branches are wrenched and broken with the might of the wind. As winter nears fallen berries give a bright colour and hardness underfoot.

Our last holiday of the year is so different at the beginning of November to the long days of summer but just as magical in the new season. The journey is just as exciting and scenic and now so empty of other holiday-makers. We take the familiar route into Welsh mountains still purple with heather and forgotten by all but the faithful few and local inhabitants and the ever present sheep. Beautiful as ever in the pale winter sunlight and with the sea glistening silver and calm, we catch our breaths at the joy of rounding the last familiar bend to see again our much loved holiday haven. Days are spent walking on a deserted beach where we are well wrapped against the quickly changing elements. One day is calm and peaceful and the next day with wind drumming relentlessly as it only can in North Wales with rumbles of ominous thunder getting ever closer. All is awe inspiring grandeur in a dark world where a grey horizon merges into an even darker heavy rolling sea as they mingle together with brilliant flashes of lightning as the elements fight for supremacy. The heavy swell hurtles over the beach in total command hungrily taking back its own as it crashes over the shingle onto the distant green in a menacing mountain of foam crested grey-brown waves, spray leaping high and drenching me as I stand far back from this urgent motion of nature at its most tumultuous. The castle and mountains are totally obliterated in thick clinging mists as all hide from the tide of turbulence, but I gasp in exhilaration and savour every splendid moment in my sea soddened state.

Rain is life giving, whether the drumming downpour that soaks in seconds or the light drizzle that caresses an upturned face. Go out and enjoy it all and be at one with the power that surrounds you.

We return home after many a backward glance at leaving the sea for the last time for that year.

Autumn fades in a haze of golden glory to be totally annihilated by the first fog of November. A world is lost in a damp blanket of clinging mist where all sound is muffled and only the occasional dank drip of moisture from miserable branches of naked trees lightens the eerie silence. Grotesque shapes loom as I walk quietly along, all alone as few venture out unless of necessity. All sense of direction goes until a light wind gives a fleeting glimpse of a familiar bush that is now saturated and sad. Enjoy the day breathing only through your nose to ward off the dirty smell of this grey world. Soon it will lift and a lukewarm sun will shine and make rainbow prisms of the water droplets clinging like diamonds from barren branches, turning the day into a bright haze of colours; the wet grass now glistening silver as the long shafts of tallow sunlight find the dampness, only spoiled and darkened by my footprints. Fog creates a ghostly different world but none the less beautiful for its chill fingers and as the cry of a solitary owl breaks the stillness, it gives me pleasure to walk enclosed and alone in its thick texture. The trees in our park are now bare of leaves as fallen they mingle with the wet grass and pile in drifts of burnished gold where the wind has blown them. The branches of the trees stark against a clear winter sky of palest pink and light grey are devoid of movement until a squirrel sends a branch dipping as it leaps about the naked branches, clearly silhouetted against the slate sky. A fox can be seen stealthily walking amidst barren undergrowth merging his own burnished body with the terrain.

With the days short and winter close, the night sky is sloe black and high with a million stars glistening and a thin silver moon casts shadows over our proud Norman castle ruins that are clearly visible, the gaunt castellations firm against the cold night sky as it stands high on its hill. Frost picks out the veins of a fallen leaf stiff and sparkling bright in pale sunshine, I step beside it so as not to spoil its new found form. Far below the gentle Priory ruins, mellow with age, nestle in their hollow for protection from the biting winds that whistle through their arches and soon the day comes when all is silent and covered in the first light fall of snow. Breathtaking as frozen music as virgin white it hides the end of natures year and I eagerly go out and let the lightly falling flakes dampen my unturned face as I look into a sky that is full of falling froth-like lightness. This first snow heralds the coming of months of chill when the ground becomes hard and hurts lightly shod feet.

Hail stones fall dancing a merry tune as they land noisily and winter storms bend proud branches from trees which were once so mighty and tall, leaving them broken and hurt until the first heavy fall of snow clings to their now grotesque branches making them fine again, whilst evergreens are bent with the weight of the snow amongst their brave greenery. Deep heavy snow that is so hard to walk through, but having perfect pulchritude as the sun sets it glistening like jewels. All is silent and pure until the rains come, making the white dirty brown and turning the snow into water that gurgles as it runs in muddy rivulets. When North winds blow with such ferocity that they pull at your body as you try to keep your balance and you gasp for breath as the howling force strikes, it threatens to lift you from your feet and into the swirling mass of small branches and leaves that are dashed in all directions.

Not often experienced for many years are the sudden violent blizzards that startle you into sudden alertness in the middle of the night with the wind howling with such malevolence that you feel the house move and snow beating with such force onto window panes that you feel surely the hurricane will enter the room. Going to the window and drawing the curtain back reveals a scene of such dark wildness that has to be experienced to behold the awesome wonder of the thick snow hurtling in all directions and creating huge cadaverous wave-like drifts on a once flat surface. The scenario is taken over by the storm's powerful intensity and mighty trees groan in their dying agonies as their breaking timbers signify their violent end as I gaze hypnotically into the menacing frightening fury. Next morning is still and quiet and only the height of the snow drifts and fallen broken trees remain as mementoes of the night's tornado. A few dainty flakes fall gracefully onto the ground now glutted with snow and an inquisitive bird perches precariously on a snow ripe branch, causing a flurry in its efforts to find a hold. The green outside my house is covered in beaten snow from the violence of the night, giving a harsh scene of antarctic sastrugi.

These are the bleak months, cold and wet but still part of natures cycle and I savour every day of my year. I walk in it whatever the weather and am at one with nature in all its moods. Every day is a day to be glad to be alive and the air is still as life giving in the depths of winter even if the cold enters your bones and causes a shiver. Learn to welcome all the seasons as I do and the year will pass with a fascinating fullness of interest and learning. As you sit close by the fire in the chill of deepest winter you will know that spring will soon return again and winter will only be a memory of a snow capped mountain and all the miracles of natures cycle will start again.

13

FAITH

Spiritual faith has to be the most important piece of my puzzle but this is not always recognised as such. Nothing has any real meaning if we do not have it. We must have faith in ourselves, to be true to our own selves and faith in a power much greater than anything in this transient life that we have. On my Quarter Boy door knocker from the ancient town of Rye are the words *"For our time is a very shadow that passeth away"* and this is surely true. I have read these words hundreds of times as I put my key in the lock and it always reminds me to try to make this a special day, to live it as if it will be the only one and do the best that one can in it.

I was fortunate to be brought up in a Christian home and in a time when all children attended Sunday School twice a day. Our attendance cards were marked on arrival by our teachers with stars and if we had a star short a reason was asked for to explain non-attendance. This was rare because we all went automatically. It was unthinkable not to attend Church on the Sabbath. My early memories are of that Sunday School hall with our prayers and hymns with the thrill of prize day when we were all called to receive our annual prizes. We would attend a tea party on the lawn behind the Church in the height of summer when a welcome breeze lifted the frills on our best dresses. Of course the anniversary that was practised for many months was a momentous occasion and on the great day we little girls would be resplendent in our new white dresses, ankle socks and patent shoes, lacking in concentration as we craned our necks, searching for our families amidst the packed congregation.

Day school always started with morning assembly and I always feel that this is the right way for any Christian school to start its day. We would line up in rows in the school hall, the first years at one end with much head bobbing, ascending to the lanky older years. As we

progressed through the school some of us were chosen to participate in morning assembly and this was a great honour. Two children
were chosen, one to read the lesson for the day and announce a
hymn, the other to read the prayer and announce the final hymn. I
longed to be chosen but was quite terrified lest I should be. The day
arrived when it was my turn. My religious education teacher was
kind and heard my friend Rosemarie and myself read many times,
but nothing could take away the butterflies in our stomachs and
constriction in our throats. On the appointed day we lined up in the
usual way and the first part of the service passed unrecollected.
Rosemarie went up onto the stage first as she was to read the lesson.
She read it well and came down the steps justifiably proud and
squeezed my hand and whispered "good luck" as I walked past her
and up on to the stage. I stepped onto the dais and felt complete
panic on looking down at the sea of upturned faces. I turned to my
teacher who was standing nearby and he just smiled and nodded to
me. I couldn't let him down – I couldn't let myself down. I asked the
children to bow their heads for the prayer and was suddenly relieved
that all those eyes would not be watching me as I read. In the
hushed hall I started to read the prayer and with growing confidence I read out naturally the familiar lines and at the end found
that I had enjoyed it. My chosen hymn was "For all the Saints" which
was a great favourite of mine. I loved the rhythmic tune and simple
words. After the service the smile on our religious education
teacher's face told us how pleased he was with our effort and I
realised the pleasure that can be derived in shared praise to God.
That teacher was to remain a good friend to me long after I had left
school.

When I was young my annual holiday was often spent with my parents, my Aunt Janet and Uncle Bob and their only daughter Jan who
was the same age as myself. We stayed in a Welsh stone cottage in
the mountains of Meirionnydd which was sandwiched between the
local Chapel and the bakery. Over the years all the local people
knew us quite well and Jan and myself enjoyed rushing about meeting everyone amidst cries of how we had grown up but never too
grown up to indulge in cakes given to us at the bakery, with a generous splodge of icing and cherry on top.

Our journey to North Wales was by steam train which was an
exciting expedition with Jan and myself always getting in the way,
but helping to see that nothing was left behind on the change of
trains at Shrewsbury for the scenic journey along the coast to our

holiday destination. We would shout the names of the familiar Welsh stations as we passed them as we sang "Men of Harlech", "Land of my Fathers" and "God bless the Prince of Wales". Uncle Bob and my father would tell us exciting stories of the area which was steeped in fact and legend. The patrician Owain Glyndwr who left his palace on the banks of the Afon Cynllaith at Sycharth, where the great bard Iolo Goch would extol his virtues to the many guests always present and the ladies of the house, to fight for the Welsh against the English. His pact with the mighty English hero Hotspur of Northumberland and his lifelong feud with Henry Bolingbroke and of how his wife Margaret Hanmer of Flintshire went mad after eating rats as she starved when besieged in Harlech Castle; we always relished this. These stories held us spellbound of how the mystic Welshman was never captured but disappeared into the mountains and into the mists of time to return, legend has it, when the Welsh need him.

At home Uncle Bob was a devout member of the Methodist Church and as we drew to journeys end we would talk of the little Chapel that we all cherished with its hard pews that caused us both to fidget, but that we eagerly attended and listened enthralled to the now familiar Welsh accent. We stayed with Auntie Lallie and Auntie Cassie and enjoyed hearing them talking Welsh to each other. We would pick blackberries and they would make us pies that we would eat hungrily after a day spent on an often windy beach and swimming in a rough sea. We were taught to respect the sea and never to take any risks – God would always help us but we must help ourselves. Strangely enough the only time that I was in danger of drowning was in my local swimming pool.

Our pride in being accepted into the local community of Meirionnydd was important to us and our passion for all that was North Wales was nurtured in those early impressionable years and burned fiercely within us and was to continue when we reached adulthood and passed this same feeling on to our own sons.

On Sunday morning we would enter the little chapel and we would whisper – would our favourite hymn be sung? We would wait anxiously and stand immediately the familiar vibrant chords were played. I never hear Calon Lan without reliving those reverent hours in chapel with my family when those glorious Welsh voices would sing together with ours. The deep richness of Uncle Bob's voice and the clear bell like tones of Jan were in perfect unison. The melodious Mae D'Eisiau Di Bob Awr filled the small building with sweet serenity as we hummed in dulcet manner the words that we could not follow. Time stood still during those inspired services when the music filled our hearts as we praised God. These memories are light years away now but ones that will last forever.

The backbone for the whole of my life had been the Christian faith, not obtrusive but solidly part of me. My parents were members of the Church of England and I had automatically followed their lead with a mixture of the local Methodist Sunday School during my early years. As a young adult I gradually discontinued being a regular church-goer until I stopped altogether. As an only child I was taken on holiday with my parents and my dear friend Margaret for company and like any two young girls, our holidays were spent on the beach and exploring our new surroundings. One sunny day that was ideal for a swim and then lying on the beach Margaret quietly but firmly declined this attraction saying that she had to go to Church that morning. I was surprised at her insistance and when she said that she would meet me later I decided to go with her as there must be something special to keep her indoors on such a perfect day . I remember the visit clearly as it was my initiation into the Catholic faith. I did not follow the Corpus Christi Service but whilst inside the Church felt a great peace and of belonging and for a while forgot the bright sunshine slanting through the windows enticing us into its warmth and felt at one with the devout members of the congregation. After that I was always happy to visit Church with Margaret. On our return home I met her priest and took instruction and for many years my welcome into the Church and Margaret's family were of importance to me. As we grew older she left the area to get married to a farmer but our friendship survives the miles and our Christian faith is a great bond. She is one of the few people that I can always turn to in my times of trouble.

I am proud to have Welsh blood in my veins and agree with them that the language of Cymru is the language of Heaven, so musical and like nothing else on earth. Everyone whose heart has touched Wales has to love the magic of the song. In Criccieth the community singing on fine summer Sundays echoes over the green and the wide expanse of Tremadog Bay as we stand together in the shadow of the ancient castle. The joy in our praises is harmonious to the ear and the heart and brings a lump to the throat and tears sting the eyes.

Faith is also private and I have never felt the need to attend Church services to speak to God. When I was ill most of my desperate prayers were incoherent pleadings for his help, when I was quite alone at home in my constant pain. As I became better there were grateful little prayers of thanks many times daily and the debt of gratitude I can never repay for showing me the way to help myself get well my way, to give me confidence to do what I knew was right for me despite opposition from people of conventional thought.

I now feel closer to God than I have ever been and do try to be a good daughter, wife and mother and keep my family together as I feel this is what God would wish me to do. I give them that most important commodity time – for there is never enough of it – we should find time for each other, time to share the good times and time to share with the ill, the old and the lonely. It is easy to be with loved ones but we should also recognise the need of others. The reward in satisfaction to the soul can be surprisingly great.

Of course there are highlights in spiritual life when visiting our glorious towering Cathedrals, with dramatic soaring spires that reach up to Heaven. Being in Notre Dame at Easter time with the dark interior ablaze with hundreds of flickering candles was a great experience. The shrines at Walsingham and Holywell also are special holy places for me but I feel just as close to God when I say a little prayer to him in the quiet of my home.

The community spirit of the last night of the Promenade Concerts, when people from all walks of life join together to sing that glorious hymn Jerusalem with such feeling of patriotism and love of God, fills the hearts of all who participate in its ecstatic praise with joy and happiness.

Not only do I know people belonging to a variety of Christian churches but those of other races and religions that I knew little or nothing about. On learning of these beliefs I find that there is not much difference at all. Most of us believe in an eternal life and that life on earth should be an honourable one until we go to join our Maker and indeed my life would be bleak if I did not know that one day I would be reunited with my mother, relatives and friends and my beloved cats. Most of us believe that our life here is a prelude to one much greater, one full of joy, happiness and true contentment, where God will welcome us to be with Him. If we truly believe this we shall live in God's heart forever.

When I was young I was sure that the evening ritual of my mother tucking me up in bed and reading me a "good-night" story was the normal of most households. This togetherness between children and parents I believe to be most important and forges a bond that will never be broken. It is a time of quiet together when all things can be discussed and doubts and fears that would always be given reassurance and a time to share hopes and dreams and talk and laugh over the days events. The evening would always end with us sharing our prayers before I was settled down to sleep. I feel that this family bond of love and sharing prayers to God is the way to start children on the Christian path and what is done automatically and out of habit as a child will continue into adulthood when the words spoken will be thought about and understood. I now have this same ritual with Jamie and hope that he will benefit from the security that we try to give him. Always remember the reassuring words "He that followeth me shall have the light of life". John 8.12.

14

MIND ELEVATION

Intellectual stimulation is a part of life often neglected despite its ability to lift the mind to the highest plateau. In so doing it also assists the body as a dead mind will eventually lead to a dead body. No-where is this more apparent than in communal homes for the elderly. Physically fit people sitting where all responsibility for their wellbeing has been taken from them, mechanically going through the motions of eating, watching television, going to bed and getting up again and repeating the whole dreary business, mentally atrophying until the inevitable end. Realistically many people accept that this is the end of their life and subconsciously hurry down the road by shutting their minds. A great deal can be learned from observing such an environment that is so well intentioned but fails to feed the mind.

The obvious and the easiest mind lift that all can enjoy and benefit from is reading. I was fortunate to be encouraged to read the books popular when I was a young child and at that time there were books like *The Chalet* series by Eleanor M.Brent Dyer which all my girl friends enjoyed. This seemed an endless series of books which not only contained exciting adventures but had a strong moral sense of what was right and wrong which is so important to a young mind. *Biggles* by Captain W. E. Johns was first favourite amongst the boys and I thought the adventures of the hero pilot ebullient and accepted his patriotism and fearless courage as attributes of all grown ups. These books were also my initiation to countries beyond our shores and subliminally became my early geography lessons.

I was eight years old when my much loved Aunt Ada gave me Paul Gallico's *Jennie*. Each Christmas and birthday she would give me a hardback book that she had been advised was suitable and improving reading for a child. This was a welcome addition to my modest book collection due to its being the story of a cat. I would read in bed and this was one of my greatest sources of pleasure and if the book was too exciting to put down I would cautiously read under the bed clothes with the aid of a torch when I should have been sleeping. On one such evening my mother came into my room on hearing my broken hearted sobs. I managed to tell her that the two cat-friends Jennie and Peter had parted and I would not be comforted until she had read the book to me to the point where they were reunited. She was concerned that a story should have such a deep effect on me and removed the offending item for a while. I pleaded for its return and she was mollified when I could inform her that like all good stories it ended happily. Many years later I was to correspond regularly with Paul Gallico. We shared an affinity with cats and he always found the time to listen to tales of my pets and to share special secrets with me about his. He lived in Italy and fed the many strays that lived near to his home. Often he would name them after my cats and this made the cats that we shared especially precious. All of his stories shone with a bitter sweet quality of simplicity making them ideal books for the young awakening mind, never more sympathetically apparent than in his *Snow Goose* which is word poetry of unassailable height. The bond between Philip and the *Snow Goose*, and the love of Fritha for Philip is magical in its purity.

My friends dubbed me with truth a book-worm and I would devour everything in my thirst to enter the soul-stirring world of the heroes and heroines. Quite by chance as is so often the way with things of great importance I read a copy of *Mystery at Witchend* which was the first of a series of twenty books commenced in 1943 called the *Lone Pine Books* written by Malcolm Saville. During my early formative years these books were read and re-read with the dedication of *The Bible*. They taught me what friendship should mean and the joy of sharing with good friends. The actual stories were a delight in themselves but to me as I grew older they were always secondary to the underlying goodness and sincerity that was Malcolm Saville's hallmark. All of these stories were set in real places that were special for him and this compassionate bond glowed through all of his words. For a child to be able to visit the settings of exciting stories made compulsive reading. Over the years I have visited all of his settings, sometimes with my parents and later with Brian and Jamie. The pictures drawn with his words came alive as I visited his favourite places like the green and white of Romney Marsh in Sussex and our honeymoon town of Rye which as he says casts a spell over everyone who comes in under the old gateways and climbs its cobbled streets. Shropshire and his Lone Pine home of Witchend nestling snugly sheltered against the base of the Long Mynd, I persuaded my father to show me on my first visits to Shropshire with my parents. In those days with so few cars on the road a journey to a singularly solitary area was filled with trepidation for there was always the questionable doubt of the cars ability to ascend to the Portway. Far north we went to Whitby in Yorkshire with its bustling harbour and quaint streets where time seems to have stood still. These books have been the corner stone of my life and for many years Mr. Saville has been a true friend to me, guiding me through childhood and still giving me wise counsel when I became an adult. He let me share the excitement and fun involved with writing by allowing me to check his manuscript and help with the running of his Lone Pine Club. We have visited him in Shropshire where it was always his deep regret that the owner of Witchend would not sell it to him as a family holiday home. I have seen his book-lined study at his home in dreamy Winchelsea where his books were written and genius burned and he shared with me the pleasure of every edition of all his stories – A Lone Pine treasure trove. Of course he has also shown me all the venues for his Sussex stories. I believe that an appreciation of good writing is the commencement of any education and no one need ever feel alone when they enter the pages of good books.

If the mind can find a twin soul the enjoyment can be multiplied and I was delighted when Brian suggested that we share books that we were both interested in. I was pleased that he chose a subject about which I knew nothing – *Louis XIV Sun King of France*. In the early years of our marriage we would spend long days exploring the picturesque countryside that we have, always taking a book with us. Brian read *Louis XIV* to me as we spent hours on the rolling Long Mynd, comfortable in the lavender heather as my initiation into French history commenced. In later years when visiting Versailles I always recalled those idyllic times spent on the gentle Shropshire hills.

We read many books of France, none more dramatic than Maurice Druon's *The Accursed Kings* based on the line of Capetian monarchy. Debonair Robert of Artois, Evil Madam Mahout and the tragic queens which touched our own royal line with Isabella, She Wolf of France. Marvellous facts which were more suitable for adults but all life blood for the mind.

Often holidays are remembered by the books that we read on

precious weeks away from normal daily life. Malcolm Saville's *Sea Witch Comes Home* was not read in East Anglia where it was set although we did at a later date discover all of its exciting settings, but in the Indian summer of a memorable October spent in Criccieth, sitting on the lonely beach where the little stream that ran from it's source high up in the nearby mountains, passed my friend Angie's house in it's search for the sea. The water gently trickled over the pebbles as the autumn sun warmed us as we shared the story of the sea.

A cold Easter in Eastbourne was exactly right for the setting of the sombre *Greenmantle* by John Buchan and we shivered with chilled anticipation at the drama enacted in the cold snow-covered country

Kidnapped by R. L. Stevenson recalls memories of Portsmouth and it was appropriate that we should share the adventures of brave David Balfour and Alan Breck in the shadows of *The Warrier, Victory and Mary Rose*.

The power of R. D. Blackmore's genius which unfolds in his *Lorna Doone* cannot be surpassed as the savage deeds of the outlaw family contrast with the word pictures of the hills and combes of Exmoor. This dramatic story came alive for us as we sat on the sun soaked balcony of our holiday home overlooking the busy ferry terminal of Ramsgate.

These last two novels were on a lengthy list of recommended home reading by Jamie's English mistress Mrs. Lambert, who understood her pupils individual needs and also appreciated Malcolm Saville's books and were to be spellbinding for us all.

We found all of these books enthralling reading, suitable for all ages. A sense of adventure in real settings with good moral standards with the required happy ending is the epitome of all good books.

As reading educates the mind then music is food for the soul. As my mother played the piano and my father the violin music had accompanied the whole of my life. In those pre-television days our indoor leisure time was often spent reading or listening to music on the wireless on which we would discourse. I was familiar with the music of many composers and was equally happy sharing my hours with Wagner's Valkyre or a lyrical Strauss waltz. As I matured so my involvement with music narrowed and out of choice contained the ambrosia of all music, the bel canto opera.

Illuminating, sometimes searing, often poignant; dramatic conflict and confrontation, momentous decisions of the soul, the hand of fate destroying the seemingly perfect moment, the running of a gamut of emotions – these are the great moments of the theatre, lyric and otherwise.

The first opera that I saw was Verdi's drama of love and death, *La Traviata*. The dramatic intensity and inherent human appeal of the romantic love story between the frail and beautiful Violetta and Alfredo was a perfect initiation to the enchanting world of impossible stories woven into spellbinding music. The atmosphere of live theatre cannot be compared with even the best filmed versions as the auditorium becomes living and vibrant with expectation as the lights dim, a hush falls and all attention is on the rising curtain. On becoming addicted to the theatre this excitation never leaves you.

Brian introduced me to the music of Bellini and who can fail to rise to the heights of ecstacy on listening to what I consider the most glorious opera music ever written in *I Puritani*.

Although I personally feel that the natural language for opera to be sung in is Italian, Bizet's *Pearl Fishers* does sound melodic in French. I travelled the world in opera. The wild arid beach setting in Ceylon with its huts of plaited bamboo partially hidden by palm trees and giant cactus which had been twisted by the wind is a scene of great drama with a high rock on which stand the ruins of an ancient Hindu pagoda beyond which is the sea, lit by a blazing sun. It is so exactly right for the rich voices of the friends Zurga and Nadir as they sing in perfect harmony *Au Fond Du Temple Saint*.

India is the setting for *Lakme* by Delibes and there can be few operatic scores so brimful of inspiration. It is all poetic grace and exotic colour in a story-book India, with flowers, strange gods, bustling bazaars and dusky maidens that ensnare the listener in a musical web. In the perfumed atmosphere of Lakme's secret garden she passes the time with her devoted slave Mallika afloat on the river beneath the shade of the intertwining jessamine and rose. The rippling theme of the attractive barcarole they sing together Dome Epais is exquisite as they almost beckon you to glide away with them.

Another scene from opera that I will always remember is the one between Poppea and Nero in Monteverdi's *Coronation of Poppea*; such consuming love and devotion and total trust I have never seen more tenderly enacted.

Of all the opera composers the one with whom I feel most in accord is Puccini. Always lyrical the delicate gradation of the music links the scenes and never is this more apparent than in his gentle *La Boheme*. Its universal popularity guaranteed regular performances and its familiarity I welcomed like an old friend.

Set in the Latin Quarter of Paris in the eighteen-thirties, the cold of winter when the city is clad in snow can actually be felt as the curtain rises on the typical Bohemian studio shared by the three friends Marcello, Schaunard and Colline. The delicate music surrounding the frail Mimi is exactly right and this contrasts sharply with the reckless gaiety of Musetta and her waltz song epitomises the irresponsible need to extract every ounce of pleasure in their transient lives. Mimi's life draws to its inevitable end, but not before the audience has been enchanted with Puccini's haunting melodies.

Tosca, the black haired, black eyed diva of the Roman lyric stage is in total contrast to Mimi, with her all consuming passions making a violent end natural. Maria Callas was never more perfectly cast in a role tailor-made for her as a foil for the evil Scarpia. The dramatic scene dominated by Scarpia as the church fills with the faithful who intone a Te Deum is to me the most exciting of the whole opera.

Puccini's swansong must surely be his greatest masterpiece. It is based on an ancient Chinese legend about the cruel Princess Turandot who will give her hand in marriage only to the suitor who solves her three riddles; in the case of failure, he forfeits his life. The scene is set in Peking and the prevalent atmosphere is one of sombreness and barbarous cruelty. This opera is different from the earlier Puccini and scales the heights of musical perfection with the cruel character of Turandot dominating the opera as listeners feel the touch of her icy heart in the music. I found the complete contrast of the background music entering quietly throughout the opera haunting me, but I never felt any compassion for the Chinese heroine.

The joy of music I have known for as long as I can remember and the composer who has always lived in my soul has been Frederic Chopin. Although Polish by birth and fiercely patriotic, he lived in Paris from the age of twenty one. His father came from Lorraine and to me this Polish French ancestry made him the unique spirit that he was, which was to flow into his music. He was an introverted genius whose music was highly individual and personal as he wrote and played for himself and his beloved Poland. He was a romantic who adored the classics, a master of the nocturnes, etudes, preludes and dances – the waltz, the polonaise and the mazurka. Although he appeared the aloofly elegant Parisian aristocrat, his music belied this and exposed his own sad emotions of the plight of Poland as well as his own sufferings. Personal happiness was always to elude him, shared only briefly with Maria Wodzinska and George Sand.

He was a tender and sensitive musician whom I consider to be the greatest composer of music for the piano. It had an artistic purity with subtle variation and nobility which reached a luminous peak of perfection and he lived in an atmosphere which encompassed this with his artistic contemporaries of the time. In Valdemosa in Majorca he lived for a winter in the Charterhouse and occupied a cell which housed his Pleyel piano. In this lofty setting he completed his preludes and to walk into this small quiet room where he spent his hours or walked in the walled gardens outside and gazed on the beauty of the scene below would have been idyllic for him had the rains not aggravated his already doomed body.

My own favourite exponent of Chopin's music is Jorge Bolet. To close my eyes and listen to the keys not played but caressed so lightly makes a poetry in sound with which Chopin is inseparably associated. All of his music I became entranced with and his varying moods can always match mine. He shared my wedding with his music and Jamie shares his name. His waltz *The Haunted Ballroom* tells me all that is Chopin where an autumn charm hangs like a veil over this tender evocation of vanished happiness, in which ghostly couples flit past and a sudden breath of passion returns to warm the poet's heart. Was he thinking of early happy days spent at Nohant where he was able to compose in the elysium setting of George Sand's home or his homes in Paris, 12 Place Vendome or Chaillot where he could look upon green grass and trees. It was spacious and airy from where he could see the Tuileries, Les Invalides and all that was artistic. He was always surrounded by furnishings of impeccable taste but loved the simple beauty of violets. He was to request them from a friend on his final return to Paris so that he might have poetry on his homecoming. This dainty flower with its death colour always gives me mind pictures of Chopin when hope and love and life ended for him.

For most of my time at school my music teacher was a gentle soul who taught us to play the recorder and gave us ballads to sing. All pleasant but tepid for the restlessness of our youth and I confess I found it rather boring. This was to change when one day we were told that we were to have a new music teacher and we were all introduced to a small slight dark lady named Miss Russell. For our first lesson with her she passed around sheets of music and asked us to follow while she would sing it through. The music was The Earl King, new to us all and meaningless until she sat at the piano to accompany herself. We were all stunned into shocked silence as her fingers flew across the keys and she sang to us the dramatic words and tossed her head to emphasise her anguish. By the time the last notes died away she had an enraptured captive audience and I felt like applauding. The tension was broken when we were commanded to sing it as she had. This I am afraid we failed dismally to do but dared not giggle at our dissonant sounds. From this day all our music lessons were anticipated as journeys into the unknown and we learned to sing as she demanded of us – the more dramatic the better. Class favourites were Five Eyes the story of the three black cats of Han's Old Mill, and often our science teacher was persuaded to add his deep voice to the cacophony that we produced as we gave the words our original interpretation and Admiral Benbow and the line about the blood trickling down was always sung with much gusto and grinning glee. As I am sure was her intention she had us eating out of her hand and we became her devoted slaves, always trying our utmost to emulate her and she could never fault us for lack of enthusiasm.

I always felt that she had a fondness for our form and one day as a treat for our long time good bevaviour she had obtained permission from the Headteacher to take us out. This emitted loud cheers which soon turned to groans when she said we were to go to the ballet. Our participation in dancing at this time consisted of the exhuberant Portland Fancy, Cumberland Square Eight and the like where our main aim was to cover as much of the school hall as possible in unladylike gallops. This was always thoroughly enjoyed and partnered with my best friend Rosemarie; our footwork was elephantine in the extreme as we stumbled through the lively tunes. Miss Russell commented dryly that we had much to learn about dancing – she had obviously watched us in action – and we decided to make the most of it. We reasoned that it *had* to be better than lessons. Trips were rare and looked forward to and the great day arrived when we all boarded the coach and were taken to the theatre. This was the genesis of my devotion to the theatre and I looked around the large auditorium with much interest, at the gold plasterwork and heavy velvet curtains. Much whispering and fidgetting went on until one look from Miss Russell stilled our tongues – she was quiet capable of marching us out without us seeing a single scene if we misbehaved. The curtain rose and I looked with interest and curiosity. I had always imagined ballet would be graceful girls pirouetting across the stage in white tutus. Never was I more mistaken. The ballet was the enchanting story of the doll Coppelia by Delibes who is brought to life. It was a new inspired world to me that held me completely spellbound – the different scenes, the exquisite dancing, the gorgeous clothes and most of all the glorious music falling in a silver cascade all around me until I was part of the idyllic world Delibes had created. The sharp contrast of the gay kaleidoscope of colour of the dancers whirling in the exhuberant mazurka is imprinted on my mind forever. I wanted to join in the dancing, let my feet twirl out those rhythmic beats until I was satiated and exhausted with the wonder of it and be part of the breath of the spirit of the dance. We were all enthralled with the theatre and none more than myself and I shall always be grateful to that dramatic lady who brought the euphoric world of ballet into my young life.

Recognising the needs of the mind was no different from giving the body the right diet. All had to be in perfect harmony and given when desired. There was no joy in reading the most fascinating book if all the time I craved the dramatic music of that glorious Magyar Franz Liszt.

William Shakespeare's plays are a triumph of the stage, and who can fail to be moved by the anguish of Lady Macbeth and the jealous tortured misery that is Othello. To experience Richard II brought to life by that rivetting actor Ian McKellan is a privilege unparalleled in anything that I have ever seen.

Words of a different kind when patterned into skillful embroidery by the masters of poetry – John Keats, Percy Bysshe Shelley and William Wordsworth are personal favourites but there is still a whole world of word wealth waiting for me to discover and enrich my mind.

Our eyes I always feel are to be most treasured as through them we see all that is beauteous. Brian and myself have always enjoyed visiting stately homes, comparing the differing architecture, the lofty interiors with highly polished wood panelling with its heavy wax aroma; vast winding staircases that seem to go on forever and exquisite dainty furniture and heavy thickly fringed damask curtains. On these visits we subconsciously began to notice the rows of paintings on the walls, always of the ancestral owners of the houses and their families. Stiffly standing gentlemen often in uniform, fully aware of their position in society, their serene wives beautifully dressed and coiffeured, and their charming children in miniature adult clothes with their pets. Many of these stately homes had copies of the same paintings by the great masters and after a while we began to look for them. The popular well known painting of King Henry VIII by Hans Holbein we often found and it became quite a game to us to try to find paintings with which we had become familiar. We also began to look more closely at the pictures and learned to understand them. We appreciated the soft velvet hat that the second Tudor King wore decorated with pearls, the rich colours of his clothes heavy with embroidery and the collar of precious stones and the rings on his clenched fingers and most of all the strong line of his face, which is how all people imagine him to have looked when he reached maturity. There is the portrait of a young Mary Tudor in her golden gown encrusted with pearls, the heavy cross at her throat predominant as was her devout Catholicism which was to cause her anguish throughout her life. The portrait is by a painter of the Flemish School and already the signs of unhappiness are shown on her tiny face. There is the famous instantly recognisable portrait of Queen Elizabeth I which hangs in the National Gallery in London, the ivory dress in the fashion prevalent in the late 16th century with enormous sleeves, the skirt billowing over a farthingale and the rigidly starched collar made of priceless lace and the white hands with long slim fingers of which she was said to be proud yet surprisingly free of jewellry except for a modest ring. There are hundreds of pearls scattered all over the dress and around the hem from which two dainty feet are just visible. Her face has lost the bloom of youth and clearly shows that the portrait was painted in her maturity.

Both of us like traditional paintings where it is instantly obvious what the painter is portraying, but this in no way detracts from its interest, for instance the famous three faces portrait by Van Dyke of an aristocratic Charles I that we have found in many of our visits. Portraits are fascinating in bringing to life well known persons of a bygone age, but the sphere can widen to encompass scenes of glory and disaster too. Sir William Allan's painting, at the Wellington Museum, of the Battle of Waterloo shows not the confidence of an untried army marching to hoped for victory, but the carnage and destruction that is the reality, the young men maimed or killed, some in their death agonies, the acrid smoke so effectively painted that it can be smelled and the once brightly coloured smart uniforms so proudly worn now torn and blood-soaked. A frightened horse and a young drummer boy survive to see another day. There are much loved scenes such as Constable's Hay Wain with its gentle blend of halcyon colours that to me tells all that the English country scene should.

One's first gaze on walls rich in paintings is for a familiar appreciated canvas. Lowry's matchstick people are scattered over his work like dragees on a Christmas cake, the unusual long necks that were the hallmark of a Modigliani, and who cannot fail to know the enigmatic smile of that great master Leonardo Da Vinci's Mona Lisa, where each nuance of his brush became a caress on his canvas. The homeliness and simplicity that was the criterion of the genius of Vincent Van Goch whose life was lived in the world of the peasant, flowed from his busy brush to give a devotion of total understanding of his chosen lifestyle to paintings instantaneously understood – just life as he lived it. Chasteness showed in his works and always he brought the darkest picture to life with a shaft of sometimes the whitest ray of light, which became the censure of all eyes, sometimes picking out a solitary item, sometimes casting a luminous quality over a wide landscape making it go on forever. He loved yellow which is the colour of warmth and happiness and maybe his wheatfields and sunflowers comforted him in a life in which his art gave him entire satisfaction.

There is a whole world of wealth that will delight the mind and it is an exhilarating adventure finding your own mind lift. The true test of viable findings are those that give a wholeness of wellbeing and satisfaction, whether it be dramatic arousing or gentle peace. All are necessary to make life whole and each person needs to recognise his own requirements and to appreciate them when they are found. Exploit them to the full. They are all there for your gratification. Reach out with both hands and grasp them with confidence. A happy fulfilled mind is necessary for total health. Remember that a plant deprived of water will wilt; it will recover when watered but wilt again if neglected and if untended will die. The mind is like a plant which thirsts for knowledge and intellectual satisfaction. Deprived of its needs it will stagnate, decay and finally die and a dead mind begets a dead body. It must be constantly fed to gain and maintain peak condition. An enquiring mind will flourish. Mind and body must be in perfect harmony. The power of the mind over the body must never be underestimated. The pleasure derived from feeding the mind its stimulating foods is one of the joys of life. You will appreciate from my meagre understanding of the arts that it is unnecessary to be an expert to derive pleasure from them. I discovered that getting well was tremendous fun and another important piece to place correctly in my life puzzle.

15

STRESS

Most people have an Achilles heel and I am no exception. However hard I try I always fail miserably in coping with stress and the ups and downs of everyday life. I am sure it must seem that I have easily fitted into a new lifestyle with total dedication and joy and this is mainly true, but when it came to keeping calm under provocation and the ability to relax I had no confidence that I would ever achieve this, as up until this time I had never done so. All these months I had worked hard with getting well and shelved the fact that I was constantly tense, was easily upset and tossed about at night in bed unable to sleep.

Of course I dismissed the suggestions from well-meaning people to try sedatives and even the natural variety found in the health shops were an anathema to me because to me these constituted medicines and were alien to my new lifestyle. I tried counting sheep and got into a mathematical muddle and was wide awake. I tried clenching and unclenching my hands and became more tense. Nothing suggested worked so I decided that the only way was for me to work it out for myself, just like I had for my diet. Instinctively I knew that this was going to be my greatest challenge, but I faced it with total honesty as that is the first step to success in anything and everything.

As I was tense most of the time I acknowledged that my whole day must now be geared to becoming untense and everything that I did must be balanced with something anti-stressful if it was to be successful. I did not underestimate the power of stress as it crept insidiously through my body, being nothing tangible but always there breeding tension and tension wrecks the immune system, which in turn gives no resistance to disease and causes a complete breakdown of health. This can happen without you realising that you are throwing your own good health away when stress takes over.

I gazed at my cat Mimi sleeping blissfully and totally free of tension on the carpet by the fire, a slight arc to her delicate body as her whole length was fully extended with all paws uppermost, showing her soft light stomach that moved ever so slightly as she breathed lightly, her head tilted back with no sign of tension anywhere. I continued to watch her often and when she awoke observed the slow relaxed way in which she would stand, stretch elegantly and yawn, open her eyes wide and slowly with stretching movements walk gracefully towards me. Similarly when she settled for sleep she would find the most comfortable place before turning a number of times and settling with a few deep sighs into a near immediate sleep. For a short while her ears would prick at the smallest sound but soon she was slumbering peacefully by the fire if it was cold and on a cushioned chair if she could find a shaft of warm sunlight in summer. It was interesting that even in cooler weather she preferred to warm herself in natural sun rays through a window than in front of a fire if she had the choice. I had always had the highest respect for the intelligence and common sense of cats and I decided that to let mine be my teacher might help me – besides I reasoned – I was so tense I could only get better.

My normal way of sleeping was in a curve on my side or on my stomach but on this first experimental night I lay on my back, comfortable and warm. It seemed a most unusual position, but I lay and breathed gently and evenly and stretched completely. I had always preferred a totally darkened room so continued with this and fortunately had a quiet bedroom. I was quite intrigued with what I was trying to do and of course didn't sleep as Mimi did, but every night I tried this system as the body is a creature of habit and I still had such a lot to teach it. Gradually my body became accustomed to my new position and I felt more relaxed with legs slightly apart and arms like parentheses and body in total alignment. Eventually I was able to relax my body but my head was still in a whirl so I now had to make that a blank. This is what I found the hardest to accomplish and I found imagining a blank did not work, but seeing a restful scene did. Often an imaginary one of tranquillity will come to mind and this is just as suitable as a favourite place of reality. These would usually be an idyllic river vista in summer but devoid of people and movement, more like a tableau, or a summer sea calm and silken with wide empty beaches and rolling mountains. Over the weeks a pattern emerged. I would prepare for bed, all the time physically trying to relax, and get into bed and stretch gently and evenly until I was luxuriating in warmth and anticipation of a whole nights sleep. I would consciously breath gently as I lay relaxed and now quite in harmony with being on my back and then in the dark quiet imagine my relaxing scene. This routine became nightly and second nature until I did sleep better and gradually as I undressed and carried out my night-time routine I knew that it was working. As I lay relaxed often I did not imagine my scene because I was asleep. This was success. It was really working and I began to feel more in control of a part of me that I never had before.

As I felt it was important to start the day well I set my alarms a quarter of an hour before I needed to get up. I had two just in case one failed and this allowed me to sleep more confidently as it was imperative for me to get up on time for office and school. For many weeks I woke before the alarms rang. I would switch them off and just lie fully relaxed in bed, warm and knowing that I had those gorgeous extra minutes to lie in pleasure. There would be no more hopping out of bed and rushing about because I was late. That was forbidden from now on as conquering stress had top priority. Gently I allowed myself to become conscious of my body, breathing gently as I awoke properly and having learned my lessons from Mimi, gently stretched with nothing jerky or strenuous – just relaxing movements. My nightly body position allowed me freedom as it was totally unshackled by awkward postures. The position of my arms allowed my lungs free movement which is most important because never forget that breath is life so see that your body is able to get the best even during sleep. As I awoke I would stretch my whole body gently, toes reaching the end of the bed and arms out in an arc and then over my head resembling an extended star as I yawned a large relaxing yawn. I then relaxed with bones correctly aligned and at ease and I allowed myself the luxury of a few deep breaths, never more than three and never to strain the body. Take a gentle deep breath and when your lungs are full only stop breathing for a fraction of an instant before exhaling slowly and completely. This will aid lung function and strengthen them generally as well as giving the body new energy. After taking deep breaths you can feel the warmth entering your extremities until the whole of you is aglow and surging with refreshed life. It was then time to get up which I did unhurriedly. Never jump out of bed or it may make you giddy and besides, your body has been at rest and does not want to go straight into top gear. I got up slowly and breathed evenly before getting washed and dressed. This went on for many months before I had achieved my goal, but achieve it I did with nothing special, just an awareness of bodily needs and plenty of patience. I now know that I will always have a good nights sleep, always looking forward with pleasure to doing so. Over the months I would wake before the alarm clocks rang. They were no longer needed but were always set as a precaution. I found that six and a half to seven hours sleep, as long as it was relaxed sleep, was sufficient for me and I always woke well able to contemplate the day ahead. This was an unparallelled way to start my relaxation programme as a good sleep pattern is essential to any healthy life and it was all done naturally and with the help of my cat.

Most of us have a "first thing" ritual and I certainly had. Wash as quickly as possible then dress and hurry downstairs. I decided that this was no good at all. What was the use of a good nights sleep if after half an hour after being up I was ready to screech. I decided that just about everything that was routine now had to be part of my relaxing programme. Washing was to be done slowly and thoroughly and with time to take note of what I was doing. I thought of Mimi, the complete embodiment of a relaxed washer, with eyes closed as she rhythmically covered her small body with firm but regular strokes, without jerking just smoothness, all concentration on what she was doing. I decided to try this. Habits of a lifetime are not easily changed. It was so much more normal to rush through washing, thinking of the first jobs of the day. I put a stop to this by concentrating on what I was doing, letting the warm water run over my hands (water must be pleasantly warm but not too hot), gently soaping them before washing myself, feeling the massaging of my hands with the soap (always the purest that was obtainable and untested on animals) and then the warm cleansing water. After washing my face I would splash it with warm clean water many times and this I found most relaxing particularly onto closed eyes. I would end my toilette with drying with a warm rough towel which was envigorating in toning me up, not harsh rubbing to damage skin but firm, massaging and beneficial. This became, and still is, my morning routine and my body feels fine. I feel and look a lot better and after brushing my hair with a bristle brush, (far better than anything else as it tones the scalp) I am ready for the day. Sleep patterns and early first thing in the morning routines are the easier as they are done when you are alone but once up you have the family intruding into the best laid plans, so I just do as well as I am able, getting breakfast in as relaxed a way as possible. The early morning phone call, the postman, the milkman and the window cleaner, all stop the routine. Give yourself plenty of time and it is surprising how after many weeks and endless patience it will work and you can relax and be in control, not all of the time but most of the time and the secret is do it until everything becomes automatic and eventually your body will relax for you. All you need to do is go along for the ride. The body is unparagoned. Give it a good idea and as soon as it finds it beneficial it will help and even take over – how can you fail with such a willing friend.

After breakfast I always clean my teeth using homoeopathic toothpaste and soft brush which was always done as quickly as possible with the brush whisked around jerkily, but not any more. This is the first job of the day. Consciously relaxing, feel the brush massaging your gums as it is just as important to keep gums healthy as it is to clean teeth. Make each movement rhythmic and concentrate only on cleaning your teeth. To do the job properly takes only a few minutes but those few minutes each day can be the ground work to your being in control.

I survey the chaos left from the night before and the dirty breakfast dishes and leave it all behind and go for a short walk, for the first air of the day is the least sullied by pollution. Take a deep breath and then a walk when the air is at its cleanest. If you have to go to work then walk part of the way.

If you are at home like me then it is nearly always possible to fit in this walk not only for the exercise but for relaxation. Walk in what now should be the automatic way, lightly and easily with well co-ordinated movements. Concentrate on your even breathing and enjoy the daylight on your face and try to keep your mind free as you walk. Thinking should be only of pleasurable items and after only a short walk you will return refreshed and ready to face the day. Most household duties after many years are done without thinking so it is easy to concentrate on relaxing. Feel your body relax and when as is inevitable you become tense again consciously relax your body and your mind and it will work. Practice as always makes perfect and gradually you will find you feel so much better and able to cope with more than ever before.

Whilst cleaning the house, don't think of it as a chore but enjoy it. Think of how spotless you are making your home for your family and let pushing the floor cleaner and dusting become a gentle bodily exercise.

When shopping don't rush about becoming irritated at waiting in a long check-out queue, just be glad that you are well enough to be able to do the shopping at all. You only have to look around to see many people not as fortunate as yourself. Don't carry shopping bags that are too heavy . It is vital to do all you can to keep free of pain and particularly in the back. It is impossible to relax and cope with stress if you are in pain so never cause this by carrying shopping loads that are too heavy or only in one large bag making you walk in a lop-sided way. Either use two bags, a shopping trolley – I actually use two small ones at any one time – or do two trips to the town. Give yourself time to walk properly, never a half run as this is no way to relax.

Have a break midday. Whatever you have to eat find time to eat it slowly and with enjoyment. Most of us can afford half an hour to stop the days activities to give the body time to unwind and let your personal batteries recharge as you sit and enjoy your meal. A few deep breaths before starting are beneficial to relaxation and digestion. The meal eaten with pleasure without having to watch the seconds of your watch ticking away will assist your body extract all the nutrients from the food and also help you cope with the rest of the day. Have a few minutes quiet time to yourself. Close your eyes for a few minutes; feel the darkness invade you and breathe evenly and gently. Do this regularly and your body will come to accept it with pleasure and just stop and think. You have now gone half way through the day and already can feel the difference from the rush rush days that are now a thing of the past and the most surprising thing is with conscious relaxation time you will still achieve as much as before but not feel mentally exhausted in the process.

Do your afternoon work in the same way as the morning; enjoy what you are doing. Work done resentfully or wishing to be doing something more exciting, is soul destroying . Indulging in negative thoughts can become automatic and bad habits are so much more easily come by than good ones. Put pessimistic thoughts out of your mind and think of the pleasure of soon seeing your family and enjoying your evening meal together.

When Jamie returns from school we have a walk together which is relaxing for me after a busy afternoon and exercise for him after a day spent mainly indoors and it is a time for us to share news of our separate days. Make the most of every time that is routine to make it a time to relax. Before long and with patience you will notice an uplift in your mind and body which will give you much satisfaction after all your efforts.

If you have a pet spend time with it. Dogs and cats love to be fussed and their devotion and complete trust in you is a gentle aid to relaxation. Mimi always needed my companionship and showed her total trust in me in her limpid peridot green eyes and the press of her small warm furry body against me. I would stroke her gently and she would purr quietly and contentedly and we would both be happy just being together. Pets are an impeccable aid to relaxation and to me give a lifetime's companionship that is priceless. Love a pet and the reward in its boundless affection will give a boost to achieving mental harmony and relaxation.

On weekdays I share my evening meal with Jamie and I always make sure we have time to be together to eat without rushing and just take the pleasure in the meal and each other's company. Afterwards he does his homework while I cook Brian's dinner as he always keeps late hours on weekdays. I always find time for positive relaxation for about twenty minutes after our evening meal when I can close my eyes and physically relax as well as mentally. This is quite easy now as I have been working for most of the time since just after 7.00 a.m. and a short relaxation is most welcome. In the warmth of my sitting room it is easy to obtain that floating feeling when you are in limbo, quite awake but completely relaxed mentally and physically. It took me months to achieve this balance but it is exquisite and you can feel your whole being recharging.

Always find time to be with God. Never forget that it is He and your faith in Him who has helped you achieve so much harmony where there was discord and gratitude in your good fortune at being shown the way to help yourself. This helps mental wellbeing and contented relaxation.

Weekends are a special time to be looked forward to as they should be an escape from routine and a time for welcome outings and pleasure. My family always go out at weekends and these shared times are always fun days. Driving in cars is not always relaxing, particularly when you become one of a long line of impatient drivers in a traffic jam on a hot summer day. As soon as I am aware of tension intruding I try to counteract this negative feeling by making a conscious effort to relax, which is not easy within the close confines of a car, but you can stretch your legs as far as possible and flex your toes. Stretch your arms out and move your head up and down gently and from side to side. Open your mouth wide in good imitation of an enormous yawn and you will be amazed at how this can help. Play a game watching other drivers become more irritated and see which one looks the crossest. Don't let them catch you doing this as you would not want them to vent their spleen at you but by such observation you soon realise the futility of getting up-tight in a situation that you can do nothing about. Watching drivers looking as cross as you used to do yourself can be quite amusing and to sit amidst a sea of cars laughing in good humour gains incredulous glances but gives you the desired result – total lack of tension. It is well nigh impossible to drive for hours without becoming stiff in your neck and stretching as much as possible is always advised. Another pleasurable aid to relaxation is to sing. Unfortunately none of my family has a singing voice of resonant quality but we have a wide repertoire and with gusto try to outdo each other by making as much noise as possible. You cannot sing without your whole body relaxing and it can be lots of fun and make a motorway journey pass more quickly.

Smiling and laughter are great forms of relaxation and contagious. A forced smile will soon turn into a real one and you can actually feel your whole body become uplifted. It is impossible to be tense if you laugh and it creates total harmony.

My favourite form of relaxation is to sit and bask in the warmth of the sun. A brisk walk followed by lying on a lounger or sitting in a deck chair with the comfort of plenty of cushions on a summer day is my idea of Heaven, feeling the sun pleasantly penetrating my skin until my bones feel mellow and supple. Move your head so that the sun falls on all angles of your face and glows pinkly through closed eyes. Feel your whole body relax as you become pleasurably warmed. This is my first favourite way to relax and makes those long hazy summer days memorable when it is so easy to feel at your fittest. This can only be bettered when lying on a warm beach listening to the softly lapping waves close by, and smelling those sharp tangy seaweed smells of the seaside. Why even contemplate sedatives and tranquillisers when nature offers you all its gifts to make you feel so full of wellbeing.

Evening should be a time of pleasure with your family or friends and to be anticipated with eagerness so now you do not have to put your feet up a physical and mental wreck, but are happy and ready to enjoy your evening . When Brian has his meal late I enjoy my evening snack of goodies with him often watching television or exchanging our days news. Be interested in each others lives and share your days world with your family when they are not taken together. I am just as interested in hearing of the office news as I am of Jamie's school day. It is restful to sit and talk in harmony in the peace of your own home.

We enjoy the company of our family and friends and outings to the theatre in the winter and country and seaside in summer. All are pleasurable and should be enjoyed to the full and at the end of the day you should not feel exhausted and hardly able to drag yourself to bed but contentedly tired and happy.

The end of day routine is important as an aid to peacefulness and I find a warm bath the perfect antidote to a busy day. I never lie in the bath but enjoy the feeling of the warm soapy water massaging my body. Never have the water too hot as this can burn delicate skin. After a bath I never feel clean without a warm shower to wash away the soapy water and feeling the water gently falling over me is calming. It is easy to imagine you are standing under the water falls where crystal clear spray caresses you as the silken water gently falls on your skin. I have a warm drink and by this time I am pleasantly sleepy as I go through the familiar teeth cleaning routine before getting into a bed sufficiently warm and comfortable to ensure a perfect night's sleep. Automatically lie in the most comfortable position that is beneficial to you. I am happy in having achieved a busy fulfiling day in harmony with my body and mind and after a few deep gentle breaths and a luxurious stretch in the warmth of my bed I am asleep.

Total relaxation I have found harder than anything to achieve and if in anyway I fall by the wayside it is in becoming tense. Immediately go into your familiar routine, breathe deeply and slowly, relax your body muscles, speak calmly and deliberately lower the pitch of your voice, no more the shrill tones denoting tension. Smile and your facial muscles will relax, flex your shoulders and move your head gently and no tensions will be able to build up in these neck muscles that are always the forerunner of tension headaches. This should now be part of daily life and your body will soon help you achieve harmony. Always remember your body wants to be fit and will always help you achieve your goal.

16

NATURAL FIRST AID

Most people have a medicine chest and I am no exception. Mine probably differs from most in that it contains shampoo, spare toothbrushes and dental floss.

My earliest recollection of a medicine chest was when I was a young child and my mother had one of the conventional mirror fronted variety fixed onto the bathroom wall. Open the door of this at your peril as it was completely full of bottles, packages and tubes of all shapes and sizes precariously positioned one on top of the other. Whatever ailment or injury befell any of us my mother always had the remedy in this wonder cabinet and I came to think of it as the solution to all ills.

When I married and had a home of my own my mother was insistent that I have a medicine chest which I duly did and she immediately filled with the overflow from her own and other items that she said were essential. Most of these laid untouched for years with the occasional use of aspirin for headaches, milk of magnesia for stomach-ache and elastoplasts for the odd cut.

With the initiation of my new and healthy lifestyle the contents of the medicine chest were discarded as my new fitness plan did not include these now ancient items. I decided on a fresh start and the items that I now have are so few they are kept in the cool of my pantry in a make-up bag.

For the most part I believe that food is still the most powerful medicine. The famous Greek physician Hippocrates, who laid down the foundations of many present day medical ideas wrote: "let your food be your medicine and your medicine be your food". With what I now feel is the perfect diet for me I am rarely sufficiently unwell to warrant taking any type of medicine. With a good diet, fresh air and relaxation it is difficult to become unwell.

I do firmly believe in mind over matter. I always have and always will. Fifty years ago Emile Coué achieved international fame by stating that with auto-suggestion the human imagination is capable of preventing or curing illness. His "every day, in every way, I am getting better and better" was an incantation. If you say this and really mean it it will help – I know because it had for me. The first time that I heard such an incantation was spoken by the character Fleur in *The Forsythe Saga* when she repeatedly said that the child that she was carrying would be "more male". I always remembered this and tried it for myself on an occasion when I had toothache. I recall saying that the pain was getting less and less and indeed it did decrease in intensity. There is nothing like proving something yourself to give you total belief in it. I know that a positive mind 100 per cent believing in your own ability to cure yourself often works against all conventional odds. Repeating "the pain is passing off" and like phrases proves the mind can rule pain. I believe in making all the parts of my body work to help me achieve fitness and training the mind to help is the greatest asset. Remember that if you try your best in every way you are never a failure. You will achieve success; you will gain confidence in your ability to control your own body and you will win.

Medicine was usually thought of as spoonsful of horrible tasting liquids, or more often these days swallowing a variety of tablets of unpronounceable names which mean nothing to you. I do none of these things. First of all rely on your own common sense and often ideas given by the wise and elderly relations, that if you are lucky you will still have, whose remedies were far removed from today's sophisticated prescriptions.

A relative of mine Beryl listened many years ago when I told her that I liked to watch educative programmes on television. She told me that she watched all the comedies that were regular features, usually only of half an hour's duration. I showed surprise at this and said quite truthfully that I thought them a waste of time and would never bother with them. She mentioned a few names and urged me to try them.

As she was such a fun person to be with and always so optimistic I saw no harm in watching one of the suggested programmes. Even though I am positive I am always open-minded to any ideas that can continue to improve my life. Education never ends. Always be receptive to other people's ideas. If they are fit and happy then they have something to offer. A closed mind is a closed life. Grasp all the help you can get with both hands. Emulate the enquiring words of President John F. Kennedy when asked why he did things his answer was "why not". Never be put off by doubts. Try it, if it doesn't work discard it; if it does use it wisely and be glad you had the good sense to listen. Beryl was right and I was wrong. Such programmes as *To the Manor Born, Last of the Summer Wine, Bread,* and so many more have delighted me now for years as they are absolute gems and the maxim that laughter is the best medicine I know is true. Were it not for Beryl's chance remark I may never have bothered with such programmes and what a loss that would have been to me. Just the prospect of one of the comedies that I now watch with such relish can give me a mental lift that permeates my being. Never watch any television programme that leaves you feeling depressed or tense. Learn to be selective and only view what I call "positive plus" programmes. These are the ones that are stimulating, interesting and at the end leave you feeling more knowledgeable, and most important, relaxed and happy. Any television viewing should be in moderation as if you live your own life fully you will have little time for the vacuous pleasures of screen lives. Never sit too close to the television screen and not directly in front of it so that any rays emitted from it will be less harmful.

It made me realise how happy people can affect your wellbeing. A friend who lives quite close to me Kath is as bubbly as the fizziest champagne and I defy anyone not to feel better for being in her company. We also share a passion for gardening, cats and eating strawberries.

Laughter is the most pleasurable medicine and should be taken daily. If you are unwell it will help rejuvenate your body and mind and if you are fit it will make you feel on top of the world. Being fit is not just being free from bodily pain but waking each day being glad to be alive and welcoming it with optimism. Give yourself a day that will produce an amount of bodily work; being a housewife this is easy. The normal tasks of a housewife give plenty of physical exercise which should be enjoyed not endured. Give yourself some mental tasks too and give time for fun and pleasure. Jamie and myself have a time in which we daily tell each other a fun item of our day – the aim being to make the other laugh. We also enjoy watching television comedies together. You will find that your body becomes accustomed to laughter and at the first sign of amusement will easily smile and spontaneous laughter will become second nature bringing with it the instant total relaxation and feeling of wellbeing . It gives relief to any tenseness and you can feel all of your organs become smooth running again. Try it. It is optimum medicine to take and you can never overdose yourself.

When you are happy laughter easily bubbles to the surface and fills your body with wellbeing and the best medicine that there is. Happiness is the most elusive thing, the gift of the gods. People often attribute it to those that surround them and although I am the first person to admit that other people, particularly one's family and close friends do contribute to one's mental state, I do know that it is something that comes from within oneself. I do not mean the happiness that being in love brings, as this can take you to the heights of ecstacy and the depths of despair, but the love and total feeling that mental and bodily balance can give. Some people are naturally more relaxed and extrovert and have a more contented nature that lends itself to happiness, but everyone is not so fortunate and I confess I can easily slip into tenseness and become uptight so that it can soon fly away. Over the years I have learned that my whole life must be optimistic and this is the first step to happiness.

Succeeding in regaining health when all seems stacked against you helps to give you confidence and to learn to make your body well by drawing on all the natural resources at your disposal and makes you a stronger person. Austrian body builder and film megastar Arnold Schwarzeneggar is reputed to have a favourite saying "that which does not kill you makes you stronger" and I believe his words to be wise and true. When you wake in the morning and lie and luxuriate in bed in those cosy moments before starting your day, think of how lucky you are to be alive on that day and make it a special one. Think of all the good and interesting things you are going to do and of all the people that you will see who will give you pleasure. Think of the jobs that you are to undertake with your best endeavours and the satisfaction that this will give. Think of the fun times that you will have, as to remain young in spirit is the secret of perpetual youth. Many an elderly person can be young when they have learned that play days are forever and fitness goes hand in hand with laughter which is the music of the soul. Learn to enjoy all parts of your day and you will find yourself filled with lightness and optimism about everything. You will become a happy person and this will emanate from you and encompass everyone who touches your life and will also enrich their lives. All around you will be happiness and joy and it will all be from yourself. Hang on to this body bursting love of being alive and the happiness that is all yours and you will have gained the gift of the gods that will help give you good health which without true happiness is not possible.

Having an inherent wish to be healthy does not exclude me from having the occasional "off day" and I immediately set about rectifying this bodily imbalance, not by rushing to my doctor but by simple methods that will usually sort out minor ailments without any difficulty.

Nothing upsets the body and makes one feel so generally jaded than sluggish elimination. The only way to keep bowels up-to-date is to eat in conjunction with the bodily cycle. This means on rising having a drink and a fruit breakfast followed by a drink mid-morning, as this is the time that the body eliminates and this is the way to help it. From lunch-time until mid-evening is the time for eating correctly combined meals as this is the time best suited for eating and digestion. While our bodies rest during sleep is the time when all the nutrients partaken during the day are absorbed and distributed around our bodies and the waste matter discarded ready for elimination the next morning. Keeping this cycle moving briskly is the way to feel vibrant. Without it you will have headaches, indigestion and a lack of energy. Remember inner body cleanliness is of paramount importance even though it is never seen. You will know by your bright eyes, glossy hair and clear skin and sense of mental alertness that your body's routine is working efficiently. A hospital doctor told me on enquiring after my father's health after his second bowel operation for tumours that all bowel problems were caused by incorrect diet. Brian who heard these words was surprised by this statement but again the doctor confirmed most emphatically that this was so. I had long thought this to be true and was gratified when medical opinion agreed with me. I have never forgotten his words and never allow my body to become sluggish. If the rare upset does occur and I am only human and these things do happen, I go for as brisk a walk as I comfortably can, taking easy relaxed strides and breathing deeply the fresh air. This is the first part of getting rid of bodily toxins. On returning I will have a drink of mineral water if thirsty and in place of a normal lunchtime meal I will have an apple, eaten with pleasure and chewed slowly. Apple is the most cleansing of fruits and gives a spring clean to the bowels. By mid-afternoon I am usually feeling much better and ready for a salad with only a small amount of bread and butter. A further drink in the evening is all that I have and by next morning all is back to normal. Conversely the odd sudden attack of diarrhoea should be welcomed as it is the body's way of ridding itself of poison matter. It is only a dangerous condition in babies and the elderly if it continues and there is a risk of dehydration, but for the average adult it is the best way to let nature undertake her cleansing operation. Never take any medicine to stop the diarrhoea but have plenty of fresh air and mineral water if you feel thirsty. After this type of fast in twenty four hours you should feel fine and able to commence a light diet. Always start eating with an apple as the first meal. This will not aggravate the condition but help clean the system. It will also make the mouth clean and fresh again which it is not when the body is inflicted with digestive disorders.

Likewise headaches caused by a stuffy atmosphere or too close an encounter with loud noise, which to me is a scourge of today's life, can be greatly helped by a brisk walk and light diet. Grapes are cleansing for a first meal.

Migraine headaches are entirely different and are often brought on by stress. If it is really unbearable and fortunately I only have these rarely, I find that lying quietly in a darkened room is the only answer. I find that conscious relaxation is the best help and always by next day I have recovered.

Never force food into your body when it is unwell. It wants

to concentrate its energies on regaining correct balance and fresh air; fasting and rest are usually the best remedies.

I rarely have the normal common cold, probably as no germs survive in my cool house but if I do the usual sore throat followed by running eyes and sneezing tells me that I must be under par to have succumbed to the infection. I always feel that like other ailments a cold must be allowed to run its course. Just help your body and it will assist in ridding itself of unwanted invaders. Never stifle a sneeze. It is the body's way of getting rid of germs and besides it will make your head feel better. If accompanied by a temperature that is obvious by alternating between hot sweats and shivering, this is the one time to remain indoors until this has passed. Stay inside in an even temperature and rest as much as possible. You will only want to drink and have as much as you need. Most people reach for aspirin to bring down a temperature. Never do this. A raised temperature is the way a healthy body fights infection and all you need to do is rest. Don't give the body meals it doesn't want. All its resources are fighting the infection. Don't rush, give it time and it will heal itself. Always patience and time and your body will restore health and harmony. Fruit is the only food suitable and nothing but nothing gives me a lift like a pineapple. Cut a chunk of fresh fruit and squash it in your hot mouth. Feel its tangy freshness slipping down a parched throat and already you feel so much better. When I am like this all I want is mineral water and pineapple and in a few days I am fine again.

As a person who likes summer I do find the cold of our winters testing and do on rare occasions have a chest chill when my whole being seems invaded by icy tentacles. Again it is important to keep warm and if you feel well enough a warm – never hot as it is energy sapping – bath can be the start of recovery. Rubbing the chest with olbas oil is soothing and you can feel the warmth pervade your body. A good night's sleep in a warm bed in an even temperatured bedroom will work wonders. Never sleep in a cold room in winter if you are prone to chest problems. I keep my windows open for maximum fresh air all the year round during the daytime but ensure that the room is warm before retiring . A cold room when you are sneezing and at the height of a cold can cause you to wake in the night unable to breathe due to lowering of temperature. This can be frightening. It has only happened to me once and it never will again as I awoke hardly able to breath. If this does happen to you the solution is quickly to make the room warm and sit as close as you can to a receptacle full of boiling water without burning yourself and breathe in its misty vapours.Olbas can also be added to the hot water. An alternative to this is to breathe in the vapours of a jug of hot water with a spoonful of Friars' Balsam added. It will ruin your jug so keep one specially for the purpose. This is an old remedy but the best to aid breathing. It is also the best remedy for sinusitis and gives immediate relief to the agonising pains that this can cause around your eyes. I am never without Friars' Balsam or olbas oil.

For general bodily aches, particularly bones, nothing is more soothing than applying wintergreen liniment. Its good qualities easily outweigh its pungent aroma as it is diffused throughout the affected area.

Coughs I find most debilitating and can cause aching ribs and shake the whole body. If you succumb to a loose phlegmy cough then this is the easiest to get rid of. If the phlegm can be eliminated with the cough then good health will soon return. If however it is a hard tight cough then this will need more attention. Keep in a warm temperature and rub the chest with olbas oil. A light diet will be all that is wanted with a predominance of fruit eaten slowly to soothe the throat. At the onset of coughing sipping warm mineral water with the juice of a freshly squeezed lemon (but not too strong) with honey is a delicious remedy. Coughs can be quite stubborn but with persistence I have found this always works. A warm bedroom is essential and the nose kept as clean as possible to aid recovery.

I find it interesting that all my life I had been a catarrh sufferer, but since changing my diet and lifestyle I no longer have this. This is surely proof positive that diet plays a large part in determining state of health.

Eyes can become strained if subjected to too much close work, artificial light and polluted atmosphere. They should not require any regular bathing as they are naturally lubricated and this is sufficient. If however, they do become irritated plenty of fresh air will help and blinking will ease irritation. Sunlight on closed eyes is the best tonic of all. This easy remedy for general overworked eyes should prove effective but if not bathing the eyes in an eye bath of boiled water that has been allowed to cool before using and adding to it three to five drops of euphrasia extract will be most beneficial for general toning up of the eyes. I rarely need this but always keep a small bottle and find after only one eye bath the improvement is amazing. Palming as mentioned in the book *Better Sight Without Glasses* is also useful. The most important thing to remember in keeping eyes healthy is to have them relaxed and in a clean atmosphere. Reading should never harm healthy eyes and bright lights are unnecessary. Natural light is the best for reading or only gentle light.

Feet should never ever give trouble if they are kept clean and when shoes are worn these should be flat and comfortable to walk in and made of natural fibres. The ideal is to be barefoot whenever possible and this can always be done in the house. Babies and children should always be barefoot as this allows feet to grow naturally. Any foot deformities that I had as a young girl were caused by wearing "fashionable" shoes that also gave me discomfort. Being older and wiser I now have blemishfree feet that feel good. Nails should be kept short and be cut rounded in line with the shape of each toe. If these simple rules are kept you should have perfect feet for the whole of your life.

Small burns need only be held under fast running cold water immediately to right themselves. Although extremely painful, if this simple remedy is followed and if the skin becomes broken it should be kept scrupulously clean. This is the natural way to treat a burn. If possible it is best left uncovered as air will help the healing process.

I doubt I have suffered earache more than twice during the whole of my life but on those occasions it was so excruciatingly painful it is well remembered. It seems impossible to rectify but a covered hot water bottle laid on the ear will greatly ease the ache.

Toothache is something about which I know all too well. My problems I know were caused by a diet overladen with sugar when I was young and in my ignorance not cleaning my teeth properly. I have certainly learned the hard way how to look after them and though unfortunately it is one bodily mistake not given a second chance for once a tooth is lost it is lost forever. How I envy sharks with their supply of teeth constantly replaced as necessary. I can honestly say after years of tooth problems these are now virtually eradicated. From a hygiene point of view it is necessary to brush your teeth, ideally after breakfast, with a soft small headed brush – this makes for manoeuvrability in awkward places – and I only use a homoeopathic toothpaste and a small amount of that only. Clean teeth thoroughly and give gums a massage with the brush at the same time. Rinsing the mouth well is just as important as cleaning and a healthy mouth with firm gums that should not bleed even when brushed firmly must be everyone's aim. Rinsing my mouth with water after lunch and dinner is adequate but the routine last thing at night should never be missed. One of the few rules that must never be broken is the before bed oral hygiene. A scrupulously clean mouth during the seven hours that I am asleep is vital in obtaining and maintaining a germ free mouth. Again I go through the thorough tooth brushing and this I follow with a clean with an interproximal brush. Follow this by gently dental flossing and you will be surprised at the debris still in your mouth. A good rinse will give you a healthy mouth during the night. First thing in the morning I always immediately rinse my mouth with clean water to rid it of any poisons accumulated from any leaking amalgam fillings. I now have any filling required of the non-mercury base variety as the mouth should only be the receptacle for life giving food – not poison. Incredible though it may seem I do know that teeth can improve themselves. All my efforts at good diet and relaxation have helped my teeth over the years become less sensitive and they do not need the constant repairs that were inevitably my fate at my quarterly check ups. They will never be perfect; I neglected them for too many years for that, but they are now structurally stronger than they have been for years and this is a bonus of my good diet that I have never thought of, but it is absolutely true.

Find a dentist that you respect and trust and always listen to his advice, but remember that they are your teeth and make the final decision about treatment. Many years ago I had persistent trouble with an incisor that had been root filled and my dentist, wishing to preserve a perfect line of teeth, worked patiently to re-root fill it but still I had constant pain and weeping from the tooth. Eventually I decided that it must come out and on doing this a small hole was found in the root that was not visible until it had been extracted. For many weeks after that the pain continued in the wound and up around my eye and on that side of my face which swelled after the extraction. I declined the prescribed antibiotics and with patience and immaculate dental hygiene the wound became clean and healed. I still have the gap as I just have a personal aversion to wearing false teeth but an extraction was the right decision as the poison was totally eradicated. I have spent many unpleasant hours in the dentist's chair in an endeavour to preserve my teeth, but now that I am older I recognise that health must come even before my teeth and I have since had two further teeth surgically extracted but felt immediate relief from poisons that had been seeping into my mouth. If you wake in the morning with an unpleasant taste in your mouth seek dental advice and if you have a lot of mercury based amalgam fillings, it is possible to be tested for mercury poisoning. For many years my gums were tinged with blue which I was told by my dentist was caused by heavy fillings over a number of years. As the offending fillings and if necessary teeth were removed the blue colour disappeared and my mouth is healthier. The decisions are hard to make but if you always put good health first you will make the right choices. My doctor arranged for me to have a mercury test at our local hospital which proved satisfactory, primarily due, I feel sure, to my making the sometimes difficult decision to have teeth removed.

I am fortunate in having a dentist second to none who is willing to give me the benefit of his expert advice whilst accepting that the final decision as to the treatment carried out is mine as they are my teeth. In addition my dentist has Pauline, receptionist par excellence with exquisite face and teeth who over the years has given me sympathy and support with sincerity, whilst at the same time being always smiling and joyful in spite of her own medical problems. She makes any dental visit a pleasure due to her own joie de vie.

Digestive and dental disorders need to be eliminated to achieve a clean healthy mouth. Good diet and immaculate dental and oral hygiene are the only way to achieve this, but as the desired result of odourless breath, firm pink gums and clean unfurred tongue are so necessary to wellbeing it is imperative to keep to a daily cleansing routine and never deviate from it.

Also remember the words of Dr. Hay "Take care of the whole man and the teeth will take care of themselves, with or without a toothbrush".

The odd cold in a tooth can be eased by placing the face on a hot water bottle covered with a soft towel or use of oil of cloves, but fortunately these are now rarely required. If you are unfortunate enough to necessitate an extraction, a mouth rinse of boiled water cooled with a small amount of mineral sea salt will help keep the wound free from infection and aid healing – it will also keep the mouth clean and fresh tasting. The homoeopathic remedy arnica I can vouch for is of benefit before and after extraction.

The old fashioned hot water bottle is invaluable and I would never be without one. They can ease backaches when placed on the painful area and ease abdominal pains and cramps.

Backache I have certainly eliminated from my life by correct posture and good sitting. A short time slouching in soft chairs will soon cause discomfort and a hard chair, or back support chair that is part of my daily routine, or even kneeling on the floor will all help support the back naturally. A firm bed is necessary without being over hard and a warm bath followed by sleep in a warm firm bed will soon erase any pain caused by bad posture incurred during the day.

Breathing through the nose is a simple way to stop germs entering the body. Try not to let people cough and sneeze over you as you have no wish for them to be generous with their germs.

If you feel faint or dizzy sit down immediately. Loosen any tight clothing and take some deep breaths, but not too many as you do not wish to hyperventilate, as excessive respiration can lead to abnormal loss of carbon dioxide from the blood. An old-fashioned bottle of smelling salts can quickly revive and any drink like tea generously sweetened with honey usually restores equilibrium. It is advisable not to go too long without food, particularly if you have a small appetite but the odd light-headed feeling is nothing to be alarmed about.

Bruises can be painful and any bang of the type most children experience quite frequently should be gently bathed in cold water which can be held on the affected area. A solution of witch hazel is also soothing and should result in encouraging a healthy bruise mark to appear at which the pain will begin to subside. Usually when bruises appear at their worst they are feeling much better, but the sympathy they generate is welcome.

Abrasions of the knee and the like, that any mother having young children becomes familiar with, are often dirty and it is important for the wound to be thoroughly cleansed. Gentle washing in fresh boiled water that has cooled sufficiently with cotton wool is most effective and I have found it helpful to use a small amount of soap for stubborn dirt. Any soap used should be as pure and natural as possible from a health point of view and not tested on animals for humane reasons. As extra protection from further bumps, particularly for children, nothing is better than an elasterplast for use in the daytime. During the night it should be removed if the wound is not bleeding to allow the air to circulate and facilitate healing.

All soaps, toilet tissue, toothpaste etc should be as natural as possible and aim to keep all the items used in the house ecologically friendly. Not only is this the healthy way to live for yourself, it is the way to help achieve a more natural world.

If I feel I need a little additional help, the few preparations that I keep are usually all that I need.

For a particularly stubborn cough ipecacuanha syrup gives delicious assistance; liquafruta I have great faith in as it helped my body fight whooping cough, even though not so palatable. If Jamie needs a little help with constipation aggravated by junk food partaken when away from home, California syrup of figs is so delicious to take, I have to ensure that the dose is not too liberal as to create the opposing symptoms.

New Era homoeopathic preparations are a natural way to treat minor ailments. This way of fighting everyday illnesses using a natural source of ingredients was developed by Dr. W. H. Schluessler an eminent physician over a hundred years ago. His theory was that body cells contain twelve main mineral salts, and that any imbalance of these salts could result in minor ailments such as coughs, colds, sinusitis etc. Their active ingredients are aimed to stimulate the body cells to balance themselves and so help the body fight off minor ailments. The advantage of these tissue salts is that they are safe and their active ingredients cause no side effects. I keep combination F for migraine and nervous headache and Jamie also finds these beneficial after long hours of concentrated school work. Combination S is also useful for the odd stomach upset and sick headache. There are eighteen combinations to choose from and it is simple to choose the correct remedy for everyday ailments.

The Classical Series are also homoeopathic remedies and I keep their merc. sol. for the occasional mouth ulcers. Arnica is invaluable after a shock to the system like a fall or bang and should be taken immediately the accident occurs. It can also be used before visits to the dentist and afterwards and I find it most beneficial for using during and after teeth extraction.

Pakua is known as the "wonder lotion" and I feel that every home should keep a bottle as it is useful for so many mishaps. It will remove the pain of burns, heal cuts and wounds, bring relief to skin rashes, stings, bites and abrasions. It can be used on dirty and infected wounds and can bring relief to sunburn. It can help in so many ways it is like magic and I find it invaluable for the bumps and abrasions encountered in family life.

Bach flower remedies come in thirty nine remedies contained in brown medicinal dropper bottles and are aimed at specific states of mind which would calm it, then like ripples on a pond spread outwards to restore equilibrium and the flow of energy to the whole of the body. From the time that Edward Bach was a medical student at University College in London he saw the importance of treating the whole person rather than the symptoms. He believed that the patient's personality, emotions and mental outlook all provided valuable clues to the treatment required. In later years as a trained bacteriologist and pathologist with his own practice in Harley Street he realised with all his medical training he still could not bring about the healing he wanted in his patients. He did notice that those with an incentive to get better, or a positive outlook, progressed much better than those who were gloomy and miserable. It struck him that disease was an end product, a final physical manifestation of a negative state of mind.

Starting from the simple beliefs that nature provided air to breathe, food to eat and fire to warm, Dr. Bach determined that nature must also provide cures for all our ills. At forty six years of age he gave up his practice and settled in Bettws-y-Coed where he spent hours walking the countryside and soon he felt his mind clearing and becoming more intuitive. He became drawn to the plants around him, observing where they grew and what conditions they thrived under and whether they preferred sun or shade. As his senses became quickened he only had to touch a plant and he would feel an immediate reaction. Sometimes he would feel elevated, other times depressed or on edge. Through this long and painstaking process he came to understand the soul of the plant. Sensing their healing power he began to capture their properties by placing the flower in a clear glass bowl of spring water. This he let stand for several hours in the place where the plant liked to grow. The combination of sun, wind, earth and water elements were vital for the successful impregnation of the water that was to provide the healing remedy. This was then decanted and mixed with brandy as a preservative. In the nineteen thirties these ideas were revolutionary.

Despite arousing the opposition of the General Medical Council with the risk of being struck off the Register, Dr. Bach remained dedicated to his cause and allowed nothing to hinder him. Because of the simplicity and effectiveness of the treatment, patients were travelling from all over the world to visit him. He was tireless in his work and because he could not bear to see any creature suffering, devoted his life to the alleviation of physical and emotional pain. Dr. Bach died in 1936 but I know that the flower remedies of this remarkable man who had the courage of his convictions will be widely used forever. I can vouch for the efficacy of these remedies over many years. His combination all purpose composite for the effects of severe mental anguish known as Rescue Remedy gives immediate relief and has helped me cope with stressful occasions so well that you can actually feel it permeate your body and in conjunction with your own mind will help you attain calm again.

I never take any vitamin or other supplements as they are unnecessary if a correct diet is adhered to. Health and beauty go together and likewise I use no beauty preparations as I feel that good health is all that is necessary to make anyone look as attractive as is possible. My hair has never been dyed or even rinsed and now with a generous helping of grey hair amidst the dark I am still quite happy for it just to be shampooed with any normal non-animal tested product and I give it an occasional trim when I think necessary. What I do do is to give it a good brush daily, not so much for the benefit of the hair but to give the scalp a massage and it is also soothing after a hectic day stimulating your scalp if you want luxuriant hair. It does help distribute the hairs natural oils evenly and though I admire other peoples coloured and curled locks I am content to be natural.

Make-up I never use. I like to feel the elements on my skin and find as much pleasure in gentle rain as warm summer sun. My skin is clear and free from blemishes and after so many years without wearing make-up I doubt if I could apply it correctly, so it is as well that I have no wish to use it. Upon acceptance of a natural lifestyle I found that I discarded heavy jewellery, preferring more delicate pieces or none at all. Likewise I came to wear more conservative clothes whose colours did not jar with gaudy ostentation, but were tranquil and in accord with my harmony with the natural world.

Keep fingernails short as long talons easily become harbingers of dirt. Never use nail varnish. It can chip and fall into food during preparation. Always use as pure a soap as possible and you will feel more content if you know that it has not been tested on animals.

Although I feel that with the average amount of common sense I can keep myself and family fit, I do acknowledge the need sometimes to visit my doctor. It may seem a paradox but even though I am one hundred per cent interested in maintaining good health the natural way, I am not remotely interested in medicine or ailments. The only problems that I know anything of are those that I have learned about by becoming inflicted with the unwanted bodily invasion. As soon as I recognise that I need my doctors advice I do not hesitate to visit him, rarely for a prescription, just to explain a problem that I do not understand. This happened to me quite recently. On examination he put my mind at rest that it was nothing serious, but that a visit to the local hospital would put the matter right immediately. As he reached for the telephone I stopped him and asked what would happen if I did nothing. He said that it would clear up naturally within three weeks. This was all I needed to know. I came home quite content to leave well alone and sure enough the condition righted itself well within the three weeks. Just think, I could have subjected my body to unnecessary upset when all that was needed was a little patience.

In my continual quest for self-healing I recently attended my doctor's surgery for an M.O.T. for the body. This is advertised in the waiting room and on enquiring was urged to have this as it was a general medical check carried out by a nurse.

Deciding to avail myself of this service I duly made an appointment and was checked for height, weight, urine and blood pressure. All was well even though I had low blood pressure. This was just "me" and had to be acccpted and I was assured that it was high blood pressure that needed correction. I was requested to have a smear test which I declined feeling of the same mind as always and was given a leaflet explaining how to examine myself for breast cancer. I volunteered that I had heard of carrying out this examination of yourself monthly but that I never had. The nurse explained that the whole idea of an M.O.T. was to find any problems in their early stages when they could be more satisfactorily dealt with and that it was as a preventative check. When I gave her information on myself and my parents so that she could ascertain any area that should be specifically watched, she mentioned of course correct diet and that the blood test would check cholesterol levels. I feel that the idea of General Practitioners having such preventative tests is an excellent idea and the nurse – like everyone attached to our practice was helpful and gave me time – that most important commodity – for me to tell her of anything that might be troubling me. Even after so many years I still can hardly credit that I am so fortunate to belong to such a medical practice. On returning home I read the leaflet but felt that this was not for me as I would know if I became unwell and had no wish for any preoccupation with preventative examinations. I took the view that I did all that I could to keep myself totally well and that this would more than suffice to keep my mind content. The nurse also suggested tetanus injections in case I cut myself on a tin or maybe whilst working in the garden. Again I declined as I knew from years of hardly an everyday ailment attaching itself to me that my immune system was one hundred per cent capable of dealing with any unwanted intruders into my healthy self. In the past when I had visited countries in Europe I had never had the suggested pre-holiday vaccinations but had never been taken ill. I just relied on my own common sense and natural good body immune system that I had helped to build up over the years with my new healthy lifestyle.

Before taking unnecessary medicine or operations that your body need not have, just think of the words three hundred years ago, on the eve of the scientific revolution, of the French author Moliere as he observed laconically, *If we leave nature alone, she recovers gently from the disorder into which she has fallen. It is our anxiety, our impatience, which spoils all; and nearly all men die of their remedies, not of their diseases.*

17

PEOPLE

Whilst admitting to be a person who enjoys and needs time alone to recharge my batteries and give my mind space to stimulate itself, people are important to me and no-one should be an isolated island. We all need love and affection and friendship and only companionship with other people can fulfil this need for perfect wellness and harmony.

It is easy to love our families and I have been fortunate in having caring parents who had many relatives, so from an early age my life was filled with regular visits to and from grandparents, aunts, uncles and cousins. I recall special occasions always to be remembered like Christmas-time shared around the large family table at my grandmother's home, playing with new toys with my cousins. In summer were holidays taken together. It is all so important for a growing child to have the security of a family. There were uncles with great booming voices and kindly aunts who gave frequent treats of sweets and comics that were read avidly and a three penny piece or silver sixpense were stored in a money box.

Life is good when cocooned in the safety of a family, but as school age begins we learn to make our own friends, often to last a lifetime and to differentiate between the people with whom we shall be happy in their company and those whom we should avoid. Most of my early relationships were with other children who enjoyed sharing the pleasures of walking on wooden stilts made by my friend Linda's father who was a carpenter when we would peep over the high fences that surrounded the local gardens to the annoyance of the people we gazed down upon and who did not appreciate our childish fun. Skipping, roller skating and playing with our home-made trolleys and chalking on the pavements to play hopscotch – all were such fun and cementing the first chosen friendships and people with whom to share our leisure time.

People can have a tremendous influence. Fill your life with those who are uplifting, happy and bright and are fun to be with. The benefits are great when two minds can stimulate each other and share knowledge. Choose friends from whom you are sorry when you have to part and whose company you can share just quietly being together with minds in accord – a shared smile, a touch of the hand, all that is necessary to fill you both with the warmth of being with someone special.

My parents' friends were an important addition to my life and none more so than Roy, a friend from my father's youth. I can recall my mother telling me of his early life dogged by illness and his gradual recovery due to leaving the town and adopting a healthier lifestyle. He was living in Dudley in 1942 and had been recommended by a neighbour to a naturopath in nearby Wolverhampton. He took up this suggestion and found it beneficial to his ill health. In July 1943, the time when I was born, he changed his employment and went to work in Apley Park Gardens, five miles north of Bridgnorth, as a gardener, to try to improve his health. During this time he continued to visit the naturopath who suggested he should try to get work at the Nature Cure Hydro in Hastings. This he did and learned to enjoy the vegetarian diet of good food. The vegetables were mainly grown in the garden and also salad foods and they supplemented their diet with a little fish about once in three weeks which was fresh from the Hastings fishing boats. Patients had no medicine but many treatments involving water. Roy worked in the garden and gradually became well. He saw the results achieved and was impressed and began to believe in this way of life. The secret of the success was "elimination", getting rid of the residual matter left in the body by food and omitting from the diet foods which left this waste. When the body had eliminated the waste products it would heal itself. Roy found that a nature cure really improved the whole of his being and allowed the immune system to work more easily. He felt that fresh air and breathing well and exercise also helped elimination. All those years ago when my mother told me as a little girl of his unusual eating habits which included handfuls of nuts and raisins I would look at this slim fit man who always had time for a solemn little girl and thought him unusual. He is the first person that I knew to regain health by natural methods. Roy is now well past his seventieth year and lives in London and his visits to his friends when we all meet are to be treasured as being special times. I count myself lucky to be included in this circle when old memories of days of walking, cycling and mountaineering are recalled with nostalgia of a time gone now but vivid in their memories and now shared with me. Friendship with such people is what life is all about.

In later years when I lived in the little seaside town of Tenby in what was then Pembrokeshire I would visit the nearby island of Caldey where the monks lived out a frugal existence on natural foods including honey and raisins and I looked at them so strong and fit and well in their outdoor lives and remember Roy's diet so like theirs that I had heard of all those years ago and subconsciously I began to question my orthodox way of eating.

I am fortunate in having known people throughtout my life who have assisted me in diverse ways. Teachers at school were a great influence and my mathematics teacher, who for a time was also my form and house teacher, came to notice me as being consistently bottom of his mathematics class whilst my best friend Rosemarie was just as consistently at the top. He tried to assist me, all to no avail, but encouraged me by inviting me to help score at his local cricket club on summer Sunday afternoons. I would cycle the few miles to his house and then together we would go to the club for my pastoral afternoons with him. I would notice the green and white of the cricketers on the field and the solid thud as the ball hit the bat and the polite applause when runs were made. It was another world of perfect gentility from my harum scarum school days and I drank in every elevated minute of it. Teas were in the pavilion with enthusiastic talk of the days play, when it was compared with the visiting touring team of the West Indies cricket team of that year of 1957 when Mr "Black Magic" Sonny Ramadhin took seven wickets for forty nine runs in a memorable match when he shared his talent with that gentle soul Alf Valentine, and the batting of Worrall, Walcott and Weekes. I learned the intricacies of the game that summer and it was only in later years that I fully appreciated the kindness of a teacher who had found time for me. My religious education teacher, who would often frown when my atttention wandered on a summer day and I could hear an envied class having a physical education lesson outside in the warm sunshine, would invite me to his home and let me choose books of his daughters when he learned of my love of reading. I entered the secret world of the books of another person's choice and gained much from them and treasured another teacher's friendship which was to last long after my school years were over.

As the years passed, sadly my large family is much depleted and some of us live far apart and rarely see each other. I am fortunate to have a healthy father of over eighty years of age of whom I see a great deal. My father's brother, my Uncle Fred and his wife Aunt Rose live far away in California but for years we looked forward to their annual visit to us and for those brief times all was full of his larger than life Americanisms that filled our homes with fun as he must be the most energetic extrovert person that I have ever met. Now he is unable to visit due to cancer but we have letters and photographs and the memories of times we shared together. My father's other brother, my Uncle Bert and Aunt May live much closer and we see a great deal of each other. My uncle suffers greatly with crippling arthritis, poor vision and is another victim of cancer and his once carefree life is now full of pain, but that does not make the time we spend together any less special. His disabilities only help to remind me to make the most of the time that we have together. All their lives they have had a kitchen garden but this now sadly has had to be discarded, but my aunt still manages to grow the most tender succulent beetroot in the world and each summer we all consume it with impatient eagerness.

Life is fleeting so make the most of this transient time and share it with others. Do not have regrets when it is too late. Share your life with others and it will be enriched.

Never fetter your life with people who do not make you feel good. Over the years many of my friends have left my locality but we still see each other when we can. At Christmas I always try to see as many of these inspiring people as at such time it is right to be with good people. My friend Margaret with whom I shared my teenage years with such fun married a farmer and went to live at Ludlow. I missed her greatly but now see her and her family each Christmas at her brother Mick's home where all the years fly out of the window and it is as if we had never been apart. These are magical hours to be savoured throughout the year and the distance between meetings makes us appreciate our time spent together.

Good friends are those to whom you can instinctively turn not only in the good times but in the bad ones as well. Such a person is Gwen who has helped me through so many heart- breaking losses that she seems part of the family. With her own disabilities she still lives a full and active life, I believe by faith, and a determination to get well. She is always first to offer assistance and always there when I need her. Sheila is another such person. Her son Colin grew up with Jamie and even though she is no longer a neighbour and therefore seen daily she will always come when I need her. She offered to look after Jamie when he was young and for this I shall always be grateful. She has the talent of listening and truly considering before giving her advice when I seek it.

The most important thing that we can give to our friends is time, something precious that none of us have enough of and it is so easy to rush about never stopping to listen to another persons doubts and worries. Remember not to live in yesterday for that is over forever; today is what counts so make it the best day that you can and give time to the people you meet while out, people who come to visit and those who telephone you. It is not always easy as you are thinking of what you should be doing but stop to think how good it is to be remembered by people who like you, and if they have made the effort to make contact then surely you owe them some shared moments. Don't fill a conversation with all your news, listen to the other person; be genuinely interested in others. I personally find most people fascinating and it is not only interesting to listen to someone else's life but educational.

Most of us inadvertently cause an upset during our lives with others. Put this right as soon as you are aware of it. It is not always easy to admit being wrong or to say you are sorry, but do it. All of us make mistakes and to admit to it makes you feel better and after such a misunderstanding a relationship is often more firmly cemented for a thoughtless interchange now rectified. I always remember the words of my Animal Rights friend Phil. She said that after a bitter disagreement it was as if something of the relationship died. Over the years I have often thought of those words and sadly have to agree with her. Always try never to let the sun set on your wrath. Wherever the fault lies it is more important for a relationship not to lie in tattered ruins. If necessary be the one to hold out the olive branch. The reward can be a closer friendship with your magnanimity greatfully accepted.

Never bear a grudge as this blows a grievance out of all proportion and if allowed to canker will do harm to both parties. You cannot speak for the other person but make sure that you do not become bitter as you will be the one spoiled. This is not easy to do, but it is best to mix with good people who make you feel joyful and misunderstandings are far less likely to occur. All of us feel misused sometimes or that our generosity is taken advantage of. Do not harbour resentment. If you try to do good you will always be the winner and the person who takes advantage of you will never be happy if causing a deliberate slight which hurts you. Never expect more from people than they wish to give. Set yourself high standards but never set standards for others. Learn to accept people for the way that they treat you, and if you feel happy at anticipating their company and saddened at their departure then these are the people to be with, whatever anyone else may feel about them.

Never sit in judgement on anyone; God is the only person to do this. In the Bible – Romans 14.13. St. Paul says, *let us not therefore judge one another any more.* Remember these wise words; they remind me of an incident that I can vividly recall as if it were yesterday, when I was wrongly judged. When at college I travelled by bus with a group of friends and we would often commiserate with each other on the amount of homework we had and help each other if we could, as we shared our chocolate and chattered as only friends of long standing can. On one particular morning we were discussing our English homework given by a teacher that we hardly knew but who seemed rather strict and severe. Now English was a subject that I had always enjoyed and found no difficulty with my homework, and I searched my bag for the item we were discussing. I delved deeper to no avail until all the bags contents were scattered over the seat and everyone looked just in case I had dropped it. It was no use, I must have left it at home. One of my travelling companions, a friend Jill, offered to let me copy her work, when we reached our destination and I nodded grateful acceptance. We rushed to an empty classroom where I hurriedly copied from the book that she obligingly held open for me. So engrossed were we that we did not see a figure pause outside the door and look at us. We jumped guiltily as footsteps approached and my heart sank as I gazed up at Mrs. Alexander, our English teacher. She looked over our shoulders and asked what was I doing. Jill sat still as a mouse as I tried to explain but was interrupted with the sharp words "copying homework"! said in disbelief that turned into anger. She gave me no time to explain that it was done but inadvertently left at home and that I would never copy any subject and besides, I never needed to copy English. Jill was also chastised for aiding and abetting me and for this I felt much remorse. She was a school friend of many years, slim and blonde and probably the most popular girl in our school as well as being my house captain. Her physical appearance belied her sporting abilities. She was an accomplished swimmer and always won the cups for our house for running and jumping. In no way would I have jeopardised her honour. Thereafter I was forced to sit at the front of the class where Mrs. Alexander could keep an eye on me and my friends on being told the truth were all sympathetic and felt our new teacher had been unjust to me. I felt I had made a dreadful start to an academic year but proved to her by my hard work that I was no cheat or ever would be. Of course in time being a shrewd lady she learned to accept me for what I really was and as soon as she allowed I poured out the whole story – mainly to have my friend exonerated, but also I hated her to think of me in such a way. Over the months she and I became friends and she was generous in her praise of me when it was merited and towards the end of our year together admitted to being hasty and quite wrong in her judgement. This made everything right and she had become one of my most liked and respected teachers but this taught me a lesson that I was never to forget.

Make the best of your friends and enjoy their companionship. Be independent and never put on others, but do not be too proud to ask for assistance if it is needed of people whom you know will genuinely give it. In adversity you will certainly find out the true friends and usually and happily make some new ones, and never be slow to thank for help given. Always give of your best to people each day. Don't worry about tomorrow, today is what matters and if you are always happy and welcoming to those who seek you out and are a sympathetic listener, you can be content that on that day you have given your all.

Friendship is not measured in hours spent together but the quality of even a fleeting moment.

I am fortunate in having good neighbours. Sim, Edith and Margaret are there when needed without intruding and who guard my home when I am on holiday so that I defy any unwanted entrant to evade their watch. On my other side I have Jane who has shared my feline tragedies with sympathy and understanding and my belief in a natural lifestyle of organic food and fresh air.

My daily walks in the park have widened the circle of people that I know andI have learned what super people most dog owners are. There is Harold whom I have known now for years and who walked his scottie "Whiskey", black coated and with obvious noble lineage with erect tail which would cause us much amusement as it immediately curled down at Jamie's efforts to be friendly when he was young. Jamie was hurt by this obvious rebuff but over the years Whiskey came to realise that he was tobe trusted and came to welcome his stroking and we all shared our walks together until his life's end. They are sad times when the park dogs die and it has now happened to many and I have become as attached to them and their differing personalities as I have to their owners.

George is another special person whom I doubt I would ever have met had it not been for our walks in the park. He has fascinated me with stories of his childhood spent on a farm and has brought the country rooms to life for me with vivid explanations of meals fit for a banquet but of farmhouse goodness. After many years of town living he is still a countryman at heart with that slow burr to his voice that I could listen to for hours. He has taught me the art of growing organic vegetables and I am a willing pupil who proudly shows my results for inspection. My runner beans are much improved with his patient guidance and the gardeners cycle is waited for with impatience during the idle winter months when we can only anticipate our next years successes. At this time he is recovering from a cancer operation and his love of nature and his garden will encourage him to become well again.

Gladys and Avril I think of as my serendipity friends. When I was a young girl I had heard from a close family friend Aunt Kelsey what a matchless person Avril was and to me this mythical being seemed so supreme that she could not be true. Years later when we were both married with grown up children we were to live close to each other and arranged to meet. When you have heard the virtues of someone praised unceasingly, the natural reaction is to be critical but it was with pleasure that we forged an immediate bond of friendship. It was as if we had known each other all our lives and we were in harmony with all our shared ideas of life. Although due to each of us having many commitments our meetings are few they are shared with mutual enjoyment. Gladys I must have known of for nearly twenty years from her Aunt Annie who was a friend of mine. A more inimitable niece could not live according to her aunt who extolled her praises during all of our conversations. When we did meet for the first time it was on a snowy day in blizzard conditions when we visited her home on the other side of our town. Again there was this immediate sense of being at one with someone like recognising a twin soul and I was to learn that she was worth all the praises heaped on to her by her aunt. Such are the friends that enrich my life.

All valued things in life had to be constantly nurtured to continue to survive and it came as most unwelcome news to learn that the green outside my home was probably to be turned into a car park for use by our local College of Technology. There was much consternation amongst the local residents and an Action Group was formed to fight for our ancient green. The founder of our group was Pat, a dynamic personality who was one of the more recent people to come to live in our road with his family. His wife Pauline is one of the most decent upright people that I know and can always be relied upon to offer help should it be needed and her sound advice has been gratefully received. Our neighbourhood is a better place for this family and Pat was tireless in helping fight for one of the most natural parts of our town. The community spirit engendered was enormous andto be part of a public meeting held in our local church hall with so many diverse personalities drawn together to do a public service gave an enormous sense of camaraderie and it was with much satisfaction when we finally won our fight and the green was saved not only for the people of Dudley but all the many visitors who come in summer to gaze at our historic Priory ruins. I was fiercely determined to do all that I could to help not only because I feel that not a blade of grass should ever be destroyed wherever it may be, but that this precious area had helped me over the years to get well – just by being there. A day never passes that I am not thankful that it is still outside my home, green and serene, to bring solace to me and all future generations.

Many famous people have come from Dudley and my father has often talked to me of one such person since I was a child. He would tell me of joining Bert Bissell's Vicar Street Bible Class as a young boy of 16 in 1926.

Bert, as he is known affectionately to everyone, is an inspiration to us all and is known internationally as a life-long campaigner for peace, often called "the Mountain Man" due to his climbing mountains across the world and erecting peace plaques at their summits.

Of all the mountains he has climbed, none is more dear to him than Ben Nevis, which he has ascended over one hundred times.

To be with Bert is to be aware of his remarkable goodness and humility and yet to realise the great strength in him. He communicates at ease with all ages and to me his charisma lies in his total involvment with people and life. I have never met a more alive person. My father is now over eighty and attends Bert's Bible Class regularly, which says a great deal for Bert's personality. It gives me joy that Brian and Jamie also attend the weekly Bible Class and I am honoured to know that Bert is a good friend of my family. To share in his services at Vicar Street Church is to be filled with peace and light. Jamie could have no better mentor and Bert's words "the best is yet to be" are uplifting for us all.

Not all of my friends are local. Criccieth is like a second home to my family and we always have a welcome from the people that we know there. Alan, who has acted as caretaker for our holiday home during the winter months, when we were unable to visit ourselves, did all the little jobs that need doing to keep a home ship-shape. Jim, a Welsh wizard of the motor vehicle has helped me out of mechanical scrapes. One autumn when it rained as only it can in North Wales, my car was heavily laden for the return journey home and just refused to start, it was so damp. The usual push of encouragement failed to help, but had placed me on the busy main road where I quickly caused congestion. Two farmers in a large lorry full of bleating sheep came to enquire in lilting Welsh voices what was the matter, as in no way could they pass me. I told them of my predicament and that I wished to get to the garage close by. They obliged by giving me a tow along the promenade to Jim's garage. Jim's face as I arrived in such a way caused much amusement. I was waterlogged, as the rain found its way through my clothes and shoes. He soon started my engine and with instructions not to stop and with waves of encouragement I drove for a hundred miles until I felt it safe to have rest. Jim is also a lifeboat man and had spellbinding tales to tell. He, his wife Beryl and their family radiate happiness and their welcome is warm whenever we return to Criccieth.

Ron and Joan have helped us in so many ways over the years. They are real gems. Ron was the instigator of my interest in birds when he made bird boxes and fixed them to our garden fence to encourage nesting and to teach Jamie to understand and respect them when he was small. I was also fascinated with all he had to teach us and from that time we have had the interest of tits nesting in our boxes. They visited our holiday home and loved North Wales so much that they now live in Blaenau Ffestiniog. Our holidays now in Porthmadog are all the more pleasurable in that they incorporate visiting them in their bungalow high in the Welsh countryside and as is so often the case, we probably see them more often now that they live away than when they were local. We shall always be grateful for all their help when it was needed, and friends like these are an enrichment of life.

People can affect our lives even if we do not know them. Those two differing personalities Welshmen Wynford Vaughan Thomas and Gwyn Williams who made magic of the television series *The Dragon has Two Tongues* argued amiably about the necessity of heroes. Gwyn Williams said they were unnecessary but the romantic Wynford Vaughan Thomas totally disagreed and I feel just the same. We all need the wonder of heroes and if possible endeavour to emulate their qualities and he admitted to having his and I certainly have mine.

Having heroes when you are young impresses their virtues on a receptive mind and I was caught up with the feverish tensions surrounding the ascent of Everest by Sherpa Dawa Tenzing in 1953 and after all these years can recall the restless anticipation of a school visit to the local cinema to see *The Conquest of Everest* and thought how brave and adventurous such men were.

A Christmas gift book from my Aunt Ada was *Reach for the Sky* and many times I re-read the story of Douglas Bader who as a young man lived only for sport and flying aeroplanes until the day he crashed whilst doing low aerobatics which necessitated the amputation of both legs. His incredible will to survive and even walk and then fly and become a highly decorated Battle of Britain pilot must make every young boy proud to belong to a country that can produce such people. I always remember his oft quoted words "*The book of rules was written for the obedience of fools and the guidance of wise men*". I maintain that they have helped me cope with all my life's difficulties when I remember his vast courage and triumph over adversity and a refusal to be ruled by red tape.

Who cannot fail to be moved by the story of Lord Nelson and to stand on the Victory at the place where he died so tragically but in such triumph, or to be silent in solemn memory of the stoic endurance of Robert Falcon Scott on his ill-fated last voyage to the Antarctic.

I cannot walk the vast moors of Yorkshire without thinking of Richard Plantagenet, third of his name and most maligned king ever to sit on the throne of England and the last monarch to die fighting to keep his crown. Quiet, dark man whose motto "loyaulte me lie" was the epitome of his life and was to be his undoing as his life was ended in treachery by those he misguidely trusted. He found relief and contentment in the solitude of the moors and was never happier than riding over the purple heather with his lady Anne. She would often wait patiently in her solar, quietly embroidering as was the habit of medieval ladies, when he was away guarding the northern borders for his brother the king. Sitting by her window, she was warmed by the memory of a tender acknowledgment of her parting stirrup cup.

The hero of my time has to be Dougal Haston, most gifted and natural mountain climber of lithe agility who was never afraid of any peak and would go where others hesitated and yet had to die in an avalanche whilst skiing near his home in Switzerland. How strange life is.

There are two more people of importance in my life – the consultant physician whose words were to change my world for ever and Lesley, the girl who showed me new ways of coping with a frightening adverstiy.

18

WOLFF – PARKINSON – WHITE SYNDROME

Over the months and the years not only did I become increasingly more fit but felt stronger and able to participate in so many more activities until I felt that all my old feelings of great unwellness I could control by diet and lifestyle and faced the future with great confidence and optimism. It was with some concern therefore, that I became gradually more aware of difficulty in breathing if I exerted myself too much and there were strange sensations that were not pain in my chest. I became aware of my heart beating and it did not seem to beat as I felt it should.

I tried to ignore these feelings even when they became unpleasant, until the morning came that I arose feeling fine and went downstairs, and at the breakfast table after no exertion my heart suddenly began to pound. I was so frightened I just sat quite still and felt my anxious family must surely hear it pounding in such a loud irregular way. For two eternally long hours my heart continued in its irregular pattern as I sat and tried to be as calm as possible and not move, hardly wanting to breathe until gradually all returned to normal when I felt completely drained. It was no agonising pain but total discomfort as the pounding had taken over my whole body.

At the first opportunity I visited my doctor who referred me to the local hospital where I had an electrocardiogram and echocardiogram, which checks by ultra sound above the acoustic range the cavities of the heart by echoes, and a halter monitor, which was a tape recording device attached to my body which recorded my heart beat for twenty four hours. I also had numerous X-rays. In December 1986 I visited a local consultant physician for his diagnosis. I seemed to wait an age in the noisy out-patients department until I was admitted to a small room to see the consultant which seemed no less peaceful with constant visits from secretaries and junior doctors sitting in on the patients' attendances. I explained my symptoms and answered his searching questions before he examined me exclaiming to himself and the junior doctors that he had heard a "click" as he listened to my heart which seemed to be what he expected, as he did not show surprise. I had also been aware of the "click" that he had picked up through his stethoscope. He confirmed that I had the rare potentially fatal heart complaint Wolff-Parkinson-White Syndrome, which meant that I had an inbuilt rapid passage of the electrical impulse through the heart where there was a strong tendency to have episodes of palpitations due to extra beats in the heart which could re-enter the cycle and lead to a repetitive fast heart beat. He told me that this was a serious incurable condition that could only be controlled by my taking anti-arrhythmic drugs for the rest of my life. He did warn me that there were a number of known unpleasant side effects to the drug that he wished me to take, including my dark hair taking on a reddish colour and my skin having a greyish hue plus others, and that over the years the drug may have to be discontinued if the side effects became too apparent. The little room seemed full of noise and people constantly entering and leaving as I struggled to take in the horrific words. I had never heard of Wolff-Parkinson-White Syndrome and knew nothing of any heart irregularities and felt that my world had turned into a nightmare as I left the room and went to the now quiet and nearly empty corridor where Brian was waiting. Incoherently I tried to explain the awful diagnosis when the registrar who had been at my consultation came out and seeing my distressed state asked us to go with him to another room where he would quietly explain it all again to us. He did this with much patience and could only suggest that I took the tablets as recommended and should an attack occur I must go to the nearest casualty department for immediate attention.

We went home with me numb with shock and terror at this new foe that I felt I knew no way to vanquish. Everyone advised me to adhere to the expert advice on this life threatening syndrome which could strike so suddenly and without warning. For many stressful days and sleepless nights I pondered my situation until the self-imposed discipline of the past few years and my inherent wish to be healthy in my own way asserted itself. I knew that I could not knowingly take such medication with such catastrophic side effects, which appeared to me to be as unacceptable as the illness, and I knew that I had to tackle this, as before, by myself.

On visiting my doctor to inform him of my decision, he was more than a little doubtful that I was doing the correct thing and stressed upon the seriousness of my condition, and that he had himself made a point of discussing my case with my hospital physician. He had confirmed his diagnosis and that he had advised me to take the prescribed medication as this was the only way to control the irregularity of my heart beat. He also affirmed the necessity of going immediately to hospital should a bad attack occur again. He also suggested the precaution of not taking holidays abroad for at least twelve months, not due to the aeroplane ride but that the required medical facilities might not be available in other countries. I felt that this was a wise suggestion which I have heeded and find holidays in this country in no way restrictive. My family and I continue to have never- to-be-forgotten holidays. I listened to all he had to say as I valued his opinion highly, but informed him that I could not accept this medication for the rest of my life as this was totally alien to my new way of thinking. The side effects which were daunting and unacceptable were not the only reasons for declining conventional medical advice. Even if there had been no adverse side effects I could still not take a medication as the most important reason of all was: how could I possibly know how my body really felt if it was unnaturally drugged? As I was now, I immediately knew when my body needed a rest, and if I did as it wished straight away I usually felt fine after a short time. If, however, I was impatient to continue with what I was doing, my body would persist in telling me to stop, and when I eventually did out of necessity I would soon learn the folly of my ways in the length of time it took for me to feel well again. If my heartbeats were unnaturally regulated it could be that I needed a rest and would not know it. I just knew instinctively that I was now so in harmony with my body that I could cope with this new problem as long as I chose my own natural method. Never for me was the state of drug dependency, only my natural instincts which were now as finely tuned as they could be, and my own common sense in recognising my limitations and living accordingly would serve me well. For the rest of my life I would be my own lodestar.

He accepted my decision as before and suggested that I let him know should I change my mind or become concerned about my physical condition. As ever I was grateful for his guidance and patience with me. I informed him that I would be cancelling my next appointment with the hospital and inform the physician of my reasons. I did this and was gratified to receive a letter from the consultant who appreciated and accepted my views, however diverse from his own, and said that he felt that he should continue to see me at his clinic if my doctor had any problems, and that he would be happy to arrange for me to see him. I felt that this was a most generous offer and gave me some comfort that he had not closed the door on me despite my initial rejection of his advice. This did a great deal to boost my confidence in going it alone again knowing that I could always return should I feel the need.

Sometimes I would jerk awake in the night, lying in the darkness aware only of the irregular beating of my heart. It would continue until my whole person was pulsing and my head would be drumming as I lay still petrified, hardly daring to breathe. It was so intense with no pain in the normal sense, but it seemed that my body was turning itself inside out – almost destroying itself. Subconsciously I tried to relax and the long hours of darkness would seem interminable until gradually, left exhausted, my heart would return to a normal beat. Fortunately this did not happen often and I learned always to keep a phial of Doctor Bach's Rescue Remedy in my beside locker, and if I was able just to put some of the liquid on my lips it seemed to help calm me. I knew that the only answer was to do all that I could to help my heart return to stability , and this could only be done by complete mental and physical relaxation. I learned to do this in spite of my throat contorting terror and gradually over the months it did not happen so often, and when it did I knew how to cope with it. I do sincerely believe that no-one can appreciate the full trepidation of this nightmare situation without experiencing it.

As the days went on the initial shock subsided and life continued, but I was fearful of my future that now seemed in jeopardy from this new dilemma which had hit me like a bombshell from out of the blue. I could never deceive myself that life could be the same again. This diagnosis was to be with me forever, but I knew that I would try my utmost to win through. On becoming calm and thinking rationally, I realised that it would be difficult to accept my own maxim that nothing was incurable, and if cancer could be beaten then this could too. My diet and lifestyle were as good as I could make them and in accord with the natural way to assist heart problems. I was interested to read that caffeine-like substances which are to be found in coffee, tea and chocolate can aggravate heart arrhythmias, and it was gratifying to know that these had long been omitted from my diet.

For a while I was uneasy about being alone and always made sure where I could contact Brian when he was at the office, and when alone for a time the quiet of the house closed in on me and made me more aware of the irregular beating of my heart. I became wary of taking walks alone and found myself becoming tense during my sojourns in the park that were usually such a pleasure. Jamie was a great help in offering to come with me always in the afternoon after school, in case I became unwell whilst out. I felt it a great responsibility for a young boy, but he had had to be told of my condition so that he would know what to do should I require medical assistance.

I became acutely conscious of my physical limitation, but still had no intention of opting out of life. The most frightening part for me was knowing that an attack could occur at any time with no warning, just like it had done on that first occasion when I thought my whole body would explode with the intensity of the palpitations that seemed to take over my person with such magnitude that I felt that I was disintegrating . The horror and fear was overwhelming. Being an independent person having a disabled sticker for my car was invaluable as it enabled me to do so much more by myself. Living in a hilly area I found this a problem, as walking up the hills to town did not suit me at all, but I soon found that I could do quite well when walking on the flat. Having a wheelchair for family outings again meant that I did not have to be left out of trips that I otherwise would not be able to participate in and added to my freedom and mobility. My only medication that I decided would help me was Doctor Bach's Rescue Remedy – a small phial of which I carried everywhere with me and which gave me some comfort as I adjusted to my new situation. Gradually I came to terms with my condition and decided to make myself as well as I could, and never lost sight of my belief that everything is curable. I found that climbing the stairs at home made me more aware of my heart defect, so restructured my day so that I did not go upstairs unnecessarily. Now, after coming downstairs first thing in the morning, often I don't go upstairs again until I go to bed. It is amazing how you learn to cope with what initially seems an impossible situation when you take it a stage at a time. Cleaning windows distressed me so I have now had these done for me for years. I have learned to cut corners with heavy housework and unnecessary ironing and still manage to be reasonably orderly.

Gone are the days of an immaculate house as it was during the early married years, but it is still home to the family and this is the most important thing. Standing in the kitchen doing culinary duties was made much more acceptable by having a stool to sit on. Cutting loaves, which I had always done, was an unnecessary strain it was easily remedied by purchasing sliced ones. Feet that up until now had been used strictly for walking took on a new and important dimension as they were of great assistance in helping me keep my heart condition in balance. Bending down gave immediate discomfort so from now on all plugs were left in sockets and I became adept at using my toes to put fires on and off. Feet were used to slide items up walls to enable me to grasp them without having to bend down. I thought back and remembered many years ago playing snooker with Jamie at a friend's home and having to sit down due to uncomfortable tension, or so I thought, in my chest. It is with regret that I am unable to play with him anymore as it was a most pleasurably addictive pastime. Hair washing which I had taken for granted was now done on "good" days and if instinctively I knew that I was not fit enough, then I went to a hairdresser for a shampoo. I could cope with kneeling down and always kept myself centrally positioned, as awkward movements could affect any part of the body, and backs particularly should always be treated with the utmost respect.

Typing, which I had always found so useful, was now restricted as after about one hour I was aware of my heart beating irregularly and a general feeling of tightness in my chest, which was the frustrating sign for me to rest for a while. One idle hour is an age when you have an abundance of ideas to be noted, but I had learned to be patient which was one of the hardest things for me, as I hated not to fill every moment with some kind of activity, mental or physical and always as stimulating and creative as I could make it. I would allow ruefully and reluctantly the keys to rest, but I was not too resentful as for so long I had not even been fit enough to type at all. A great disappointment was an inability to be as active in the garden as I was formerly. I now do the lighter jobs and still take pleasure in weeding on a summer day when the warmth of the sun envelopes me and helps ease general tension. Growing plants and vegetables I still participate in and with plenty of help and some encouragement life continued. Walking was still pleasurable but standing still aggravated my condition. When in the park there were plenty of strategically placed benches and in summer many people to sit with and give me their welcome company. In winter or rain I still needed a short time to sit down but I got many a curious look as I sat in the rain. I had learned not to mind and actually enjoyed any weather and was glad I was able to walk at all as I still considered myself fortunate to be alive with such a lot stacked against me. I do believe in luck, and luck ensured that I had survived two car crashes and many scary moments that were not of my doing and not in my control, but so much of our lives we can control and I make sure I give my body all the help that I can at all times.

I had always enjoyed the company of friends and relatives and entertaining at home and vice versa had for as long as I could remember been a part of my social life. It was with distress that I found that after participating in this, no matter how relaxed and enjoyable, after about an hour I would notice the commencement of an irregular heart beat, and if I continued for even less that two hours of the most welcome companionship I was acutely miserable and quite unable to concentrate on the chatter and laughter, my only awareness being of my growing discomforture. After this had happened on a number of occasions I realised that talking was the main culprit and for me to continue any sort of social activity this had to be monitored. In no way did I not wish to see the people that I cared for, so Brian and I decided to curtail visits to see if it helped. This certainly did, and after usually an hour and a half when I found that my heart told me that it had had enough, most people were sympathetic and understanding and so I was able to continue to enjoy my visitors for short durations. If I overdid it then I was the one to suffer, often for days before my heart would settle into a regular pattern. Our life was then enhanced by the people who understood that late nights were now out for me. Theatre visits I was relieved to find could be undertaken with no adverse problems, probably due to me not having actively to participate, but only sit back and see the story unfolding on the stage. I was no hedonist, but from now on all pleasure took on a new meaning and the struggle to obtain it made it more gratifying .

I learned and accepted my limitations as in no way would I knowingly allow myself to be on a collision course to disaster and often I have heard of people talk of the quality of life. Well forget it. When you are in danger of losing it then all you want is to survive – the quality can be gained later. Years ago when I felt so ill I had never wanted to die and now that I felt so much better and stronger generally, the will to survive was even more pronounced. People who talk of the quality of life are usually fit and feel in no danger of losing theirs. Give up hope and you will die anyway. Fight and you are half way to winning and perseverance will see that you will. Always keep your spirits up and never give in. I was not going to give up ever, and I was truly happy even in my restricted state, because I knew that as I learned more of the cause of my condition then I could rectify it. My aim of total wellness would be achieved and only this would I consider the ultimate goal. Never let anyone stop you in your travail for life's most glittering prize – good health.

Even though I adapted as well as I could and never regretted forsaking medication for the rest of my life – which I wished to be lengthy and healthy – I still felt so alone as no-one seemed to have heard of my condition. I often felt wistfully that if I could talk to someone who also had these strange feelings and sensations that were not really pain but the knowledge that a vital part of your body was malfunctioning, I would not be so isolated. In November 1987 when I felt that I had made great strides in sorting out my life as well as I could, I turned a page in the local newspaper that I was reading to find a headline in large letters that caught my attention with the photograph of a young girl beneath it. I started idly to read it until my whole attention was captured as if hypnotised as I followed the story of a twelve year old Oldbury girl Sonia Reading who had Wolf-Parkinson-White Syndrome. My first reaction was of such relief to find a fellow sufferer, and as it appeared she had had this from birth and had received orthodox treatment, I felt sure that it would help to talk to her. Her mother had been aware immediately that her daughter's heart was beating fast and during her childhood she had been hospitalised more than fifty times when it was not possible to treat her at home. Her father told me that she had to take medication daily to control her heartbeat, but that in August 1988 she was to visit the Brompton Hospital in Kensington, London for tests prior to an operation in a bid to cure her of the condition. After the visit her mother said that the staff at the hospital were reassuring and had every confidence that they could give Sonia a total cure and that this was the best news that they had had in a long time. In October 1988, Sonia returned to Brompton Hospital for a laser treatment where surgeons tried to discover the nerves which made her heart suddenly beat up to two hundred times a second. Originally they thought they had failed to block some of them but later realised their success when Sonia's heartbeat became normal. I was delighted at this news for Sonia for I knew from her father how she had tried to keep up with her school studies and not let her heart abnormality stop her from leading a normal life. It was with bitter disappointment for her that she told me later that the laser treatment had only lasted for a few months and not been a success and that the old condition had returned, necessitating her to resume daily medication to regulate her heartbeat. I hope that some day this brave girl will be helped as she has her own whole life ahead of her and I wish her all success in mathematics and banking should her interest continue in this direction. When I talked to Sonia's father I told him how I was treating my condition with change of lifestyle and diet and he said that he understood how I felt and maybe that I could have the answer. The lack of success for Sonia has only made me more determined to continue to try to cure myself. The best orthodox medical treatment had been unable to help Sonia so I reasoned that I had helped myself quite miraculously over the past years and saw no reason why I could not do so again.

I felt buoyant to be doing something positive, so it was back to the drawing board to learn all that I could about any irregular heart conditions that would help me. As a person of no medical knowledge and no interest in anything medical I really had to start from the bottom, as I was quite ignorant of most bodily functions unless I had to find out the hard way by becoming a victim. I felt like a pioneer as I read all that I could to try to find a pattern of what had caused my heart initially to malfunction, so that I could put right my mistake and when I found it there would be no retrograde steps. I still believe that we are all responsible for our state of health and first I would find this cause and then find the diet most suited to help me. I knew that my diet was excellent and with its anti-cancer foods could not be bettered as a general basis, but I knew also that there was something that I was missing due to ignorance. So with patience and lots of research from all the sources that I could find I decided to find a cure in my own way, not to be tried out on poor defenceless animals but the real live guinea pig – me. I still had total faith in all I was doing and was eager to experiment on myself and monitor the results. I still had every intention of walking positively into life with arms outstretched to encompass all that was good and I could only do this if my whole body was in perfect balance with optimum fitness.

Instinctively I knew that finding out all that I could about my medical condition would be the hardest, so I decided to tackle this first. Mentally I tried to help myself by putting everything into perspective. This was a setback that was part of my whole. I must not fall into the trap of thinking of just a heart abnormality. My heart was part of me and I must help the whole of me which in turn would help my heart. I had proved to myself that I could with patience and determination cure illness. There was no reason why I could not cure this. This was another challenge, a new one that I would face head on and win.

I could find little in my local libraries about Wolff-Parkinson-White Syndrome so I decided to concentrate on anything that seemed similar to it as I reasoned that whatever medical name was given, any malfunction of the electrical system in the heart could probably be caused by some factor that was familiar in many cases. For months I felt I was groping in the dark without finding anything that I recognised would be of substance to help me, until I happened to read of Sudden Unexplained Death Syndrome, which was fully explained in a British Broadcasting Corporation Television *Horizon* programme. This apparently killed hundreds of thousands of people worldwide each year and every year; sudden death is a major scourge in the United Kingdom and kills between 50,000 and 100,000 Britons every year. In the Unites States that figure was a quarter of a million which means there are victims every 60 to 90 seconds. Many of these victims had some history of coronary heart disease but it was not the classic heart attack that killed but a rapid onset of fatal electrical activity in the heart.these last words were what captured my attention as this was exactly the condition of Wolff-Parkinson-White Syndrome which from what my consultant had told me could be just as fatal if the heartbeat did not return to its correct rhythm.

I drank in this new found knowledge as one dying of thirst and with growing excitement that I had discovered something of great importance to me of how an apparently healthy person with no obvious heart defects could become a victim of sudden death due to the hearts electrical instability. Perplexingly, sudden cardiac death remains a major killer yet it gains hardly any attention. It gained little recognition probably because it was out of sight and out of mind. Death was clean, you're gone, no lingering death that could be observed over months or even years. Knowing nothing of medical knowledge of the heart I was relieved that even a lay person such as myself had no difficulty in comprehending the easily understood words. The heart is a four chambered pump that is driven and synchronised by electricity. Pulses from the heart's own pacemaker produce a smooth rhythm of contraction and relaxation. However, after a heart attack, a myo-cardial infarction, which has killed or damaged a small area of the heart muscle, the electrical impulses travel at normal speeds through the undamaged tissue but the conduction speed in the infarcted area is much reduced. Suddenly, a fast rotating current, called re-entry , can spontaneously form. It rapidly spreads to complete disorganisation. This is one pathway to ventricular fibrillation – sudden death. It was not necessary to be a heart attack sufferer to fibrillate and all of this was so similar to what had been explained to me of Wolff-Parkinson-White Syndrome that I continued to read, not so much as to gain medical knowledge in a general sense, but only to try to educate myself so that I could help my own condition which seemed to run parallel with this one.

I read the findings of Dr. Stewart Wolf who had been monitoring the ages and causes of death of the citizens of Roseto, an Italian community in North-East Pennsylvania for over twenty years. These people appeared to eat all of the wrong foods attributed to contributing to heart diseases. They were fat and liked to smoke and drink and on physical examination were shown to be healthy people. It was amazing that when examining someone eighty five years old, nothing could be found wrong with him. It appeared that the secret of survival was that the whole town had grown up steadily from the descendants of nineteenth century settlers into a community comprised of tightly-knit extended families, or clans. This social structure was still much alive in the 1950s when Dr. Wolf started his research, but by the early 1960s the younger generation were already showing signs of deserting the old social values and Dr. Wolf predicted that as they did so they would lose their immunity to heart disease. This proved to be the case as even though these younger generations were more aware of eating less fat and smoking less, they were dying in greater numbers. Dr. Wolf believed that the power of clan protects against death from heart disease. His hypothesis pointed to the value of traditional, supportive social networks in lowering stress. When these were absent heart trouble could be expected. This was a sobering revelation to me as coping with stress had always been the problem I had found hardest to overcome. The easiest thing in the world for me to do was to become "keyed up" and "nervy" and this immediately upset my heart and would cause palpitations. The nerves, the autonomic nervous system that linked the brain to the heart was composed of two branches, both of which connected to the heart's main pacemaker. The sympathetic nerve releases adrenalin and speeds up the heart; but the vagus nerve is dominant and slows it down. Both these nervous systems have projections directly to the ventricles of the heart. Here the sympathetic nerve is dominant and adrenalin can electrically destabilise the heart. Stress could cause sudden death so nervous input to the heart was necessary for it to occur. It could be news of a disaster or just as easily happy news, either way it could give a shock to the nervous input and be fatal.

I learned of the long QT syndrome, where the slightest shock can kill, even though there is no heart disease. On an electrocardiograph each bit of the cardiac cycle is assigned a letter. The QRS is when the ventricles contract and the T-wave is when they recharge before contracting again, but in long QT syndrome the T-wave is drawn out. The enlarged distance between the Q and the T is a sign of electrical instability. All of these attacks were triggered by emotional conditions, or by physical stress and under these conditions it was known that a major discharge in the sympathetic nervous system occurred towards the heart. The sympathetic nerve supply to the heart has two branches and it is believed that in long QT sufferers the left sided nerves are dominant. Release of adrenalin throughout the heart was, therefore, very uneven. This release into the heart in a non-uniform manner could contribute to lethal arrhythmias. It could start when faced with first emotions whilst playing with other children and family troubles. It was under these conditions of stress or physical exercise that there could be syncopal attacks. Syncopy was basically a transient cardiac arrest that leads to a complete loss of blood pressure and therefore the patient basically faints. The long QT interval is now used as a warning sign of a heart in danger of arrhythmia, whatever the disease background. It clearly implicates the role of the sympathetic nerve in triggering sudden death. It was known that when the heart became starved of oxygen a shock reaction excited the sympathetic nerve and caused the heart to race. This stressed the heart still further. However, it was noted that when blood pressure rises inside the arteries it could stimulate the vagus nerve which compensated by slowing the heart down. This showed that whilst the sympathetic nerve could cause sudden death, the vagus nerve, if it was robust enough, could prevent it. Most of these deaths were caused at night when patients were asleep and should have been relaxed and usually in their homes, entirely free of any stress of daily life. This all made sense to me because if you had stress in the day you could sleep out of exhaustion and if your mind was not at rest the body would continue to be stressed. I thought of how when my condition had first been diagnosed in the following weeks I would wake in the middle of the night from a comparatively peaceful sleep to be aware of my heart beating irregularly. It was so intense that it had woken me. I would lie awake in the dark and be aware of the uneven beats pounding through my body until the whole of me seemed an irregular pulse. Subconsciously I had tried to relax and my years of discipline had overcome my terror until the uneven heart beat subsided. Sometimes Brian would sit beside me unable to help but I did derive some comfort from his presence and when I asked him to feel my heartbeat he said that he could easily feel it racing haphazardly. Most of the time I just coped by myself as I could see no point in waking and worrying him for no purpose. This was the nearest that I had ever come to identifying something that was so like mine. It is so difficult to explain something that you do not understand and it was with tremendous relief that I learned that what I had – or something similar to it – was so common. What I wanted to do was put all the fragments together to form a clear picture so that I could learn to help myself more.

I read on, always learning and always looking for some correlation between health and diet, as I believed implicitly that this was the key to all illness and over the years I had now proved this to be so – it just had to be the same with this heart condition – and then I found it. The consanguinity law did prevail as blood tests had shown that a large proportion of people at high risk with a heart in danger of arrhythmia were found to be low in thiamine; this was vitamin B1 which could be derived from food. The main task of thiamine is to help convert carbohydrate foods into energy, but it also keeps nerves healthy, especially those of the heart. Too little thiamine could bring on depression and irritability; severe deficiency hits the whole body and leads to beri-beri which affects nerves and muscle power and causes heart failure. It is needed for energy production, growth, appetite, digestion and helps the breakdown of carbohydrate, protein and fat to release energy. Our bodies cannot store the B vitamins for long so a daily supply was important. These medical tests proved the affiliation between diet and subsequent heart damage. In America a dietary expert had conducted experiments where people were put on a diet from which all thiamine had been excluded, and the subjects were exercised on treadmills and tests of their autonomic function, including electrocardiographs were regularly taken. Within two weeks they showed a lengthening of the QT interval in the test. The vitamin deficiency had put their hearts in danger of arrhythmia. They were given vitamin tablets and the electrocardiographs returned to normal. This proved to me beyond any doubt whatsoever that I was completely correct in my belief that diet – and only correctly balanced diet – held the key to cessation of health defects. I checked to see whether my diet had an adequate supply of thiamine. The richest natural sources of this vitamin were to be found in yeast, wholegrains, pork, liver, nuts, legumes, potatoes, soya beans, bread and flour, peas, beans, lentils, milk, eggs, molasses, many seeds (especially sprouting ones), fish, fruit and cereals. I was amazed at the list and immediately decided to step up my intake of this vitamin. I certainly had this valuable B1 in my diet and was particularly interested to read that sunflower seeds were an excellent source of vital nutrients. They contained most of the B vitamins, vitamin E and also many essential fatty acids, and pound for pound twice as much iron and twenty five times as much thiamine as steak. In addition sunflower seeds also had a mildly soothing, sedative effect on the nervous system as they contained various sedative essential oils. Sunflower seeds also stimulated the adrenal glands and of course were non-allergic. These little gems must surely figure more in my diet. I had always enjoyed them and their sweet nutty flavour was an ideal cooked meal combination with many vegetables. I particularly savoured a plate of them with lightly steamed cauliflower. Sprouted they rivalled meat in nutritive value and were the richest source of naturally occurring vitamins known and also contained an excellent balance of amino acids, fatty acids and natural sugars, plus a high content of minerals. They have been recognised as high quality food for almost 5000 years and references to them were found in documents written at the time of Jesus. They are an important part of the diet of the long lived Hunza people of the Himalayas. The vitamin content of seeds increases phenomenally when they germinate and in sprouted wheat the thiamine increases by 30 per cent. I decided to include more of these sprouts plus lentils, sunflower seeds and pumpkin seeds into my diet as they were often overlooked when I just forgot to prepare them. Of all the other food items rich in so many nutrients as well as this important thiamine I just decided to step up the amount of suitable foods already in my diet. It was all so simple to do when knowing the direction to go and yet as in so many important things I only read of this quite by chance. My panacea for all bodily imbalance was need for dietary correction and to achieving correct equilibrium in my diet which I could easily and with much pleasure accomplish. To cognate this with stress control which was equally important I would find much harder, but I intended to succeed, I had to, my life could depend on it.

I visited my doctor and explained to him what I had found out and he checked in his medical books and read to me that vitamin B deficiency was usually found in alcoholics and people with poor diet. This was amusing as I never touched alcohol and was quite content with my good diet. He said that he would check the matter with the local hospital who also confirmed what he had told me, that if I had a good varied diet I would not be short of any vitamins. This is what I had long felt myself and he did volunteer that he grew his own vegetables as even when buying fresh food you could never be sure that they had not been sprayed with some chemical, unless you were able to purchase organic produce. He said that the slugs had a healthy appetite for his home grown food and felt that this could not be bad, you just needed extra scrutiny of the food before consuming it. As I had found that slugs were of the highest intelligence and they only consumed the choicest of my own garden goodies, I agreed with what he said. I pondered on my doctors words as I had much regard for him and his common sense attitude in helping me. I felt that he was right in that my diet was fine as it was, but I knew myself that everything in life can always be bettered, so intended to rebalance my diet so that the foods that contained thiamine that I already ate with pleasure would from now on be eaten in larger quantities. It was just so easy to have an extra nut meal, more peas and beans, a spoon of thick molasses on my porridge and more sprouted seeds. I knew that it would all help. On reflection I realised that although I had eaten correctly for many years, for a long time this had not been so. I had had many years of stress, a heavy workload and a poor diet when I had been so tired and I had often missed meals altogether. I had become disorientated at the deaths prematurely of people that I cared for and over the years I had not been able to come to terms with it. This had given me the same heart stress as Sudden Death Syndrome victims. This downward spiral had contributed to my pitiful condition of all those years ago and could have been the commencement of my heart problems. The more I considered it the more I thought that I had totally but uncon-sciously brought about my own heart condition, but like so many bodily imbalances it had taken many years before it had become apparent. This cheered me tremendously as I always now had to have the right answers and the whole answers to any problem and then I could go forward and put things right. In this case I was fortunate in having my doctor help me, and when he sug-gested that I have a general blood test taken I readily agreed, and when this proved satisfactory I turned with confidence and renewed interest in restructuring my diet so that it was as full of curative goodness as I could make it.

All these findings proved that electrical instability in the heart could be caused by low thiamine levels in the blood, poor general nutrition and a high level of stress. It was a potentially lethal combination. Some extra factor, possibly genetic, possibly unknown, could single out susceptible individuals. Then subtle damage to their hearts, or autonomic nervous system, did the rest and stress pulled the trigger. It proved that Sudden Death could occur against a background of poverty or against a background of affluence. I intended to do all that I could to see that I did not become a Sudden Death statistic.

As vitamin E had always been recommended for good heart function generally in all the health books that I had read, I refreshed my memory about this major antioxidant which was vital for health of blood vessels and protected the cells from the harmful effect of too much oxygen. It prevented blood clots and was needed for growth and repair of skin, particularly after wounding, and promoted healthy muscles. Vitamin E is stored in the body and it was interesting to note that this could be depleted by a high intake of polyunsaturated oils and fats – as recommended by doctors to help prevent heart disease – and this made me able to enjoy the delights of butter even more. Air pollution could also destroy this vitamin but I was confident that I did all that I could to live in an unpolluted atmosphere. The richest natural sources were vegetable oils, fish oils, wheatgerm, leafy vegetables, egg yolk, legumes, lettuce, peanuts, wholewheat flour and a variety of seeds so I was satisfied that I could consume an adequate daily supply when it could be found in so much of my usual diet.

The mineral selenium was also known to protect the heart generally and also worked with vitamin E to protect body tissues from aging and to resist infection. It is named after Selene, the Goddess of the Moon, and is part of the earth's every fabric. Where it is found in the soil, it is usually part of volcanic ash produced by prehistoric volcanoes, but years of chemical farming methods, destruction of topsoil and overplanting have left many farmlands denuded of selenium – just as its nutritional value is becoming more widely understood. Its role as a nutrient was first identified in the 1950s. Studies on humans have shown that consuming adequate selenium seemed to lessen the likelihood of developing cancer as well as protecting the heart. It is a semi-metallic element which in tiny, crucial amounts, is an essential nutrient of the human diet. The amount of selenium in food is dependent on the richness of the soil. Its distribution around the world is irregular – abundant in some areas, negligible in others. The levels in the United Kingdom are generally low although there are some high areas such as Norfolk, which has a selenium-rich soil.

The mineral's importance derives mainly from the protection it gives against the effect of oxygen on the body's tissues. It is a major component of one of our most important antioxidant enzymes. Although we depend on oxygen for life itself, it also has a destructive side and without adequate protective agents like selenium, it causes disease and accelerates ageing. Its harmful action is exacerbated by every facet of unhealthy living, from alcohol to pollution. Oxygen is the major cause of the damage to molecules which makes them into free radicals – harmful, disease causing elements wreaking havoc in the body. Free radicals continue reproducing themselves and it is selenium's antioxidant effect on this whole process which underlies the numerous vital ways in which the body makes use of it.

The richest natural sources were fish – tuna is particularly good; yeast, whole grains, brown rice, organ meats, eggs, onions and garlic, mushrooms, asparagus, broccoli and tomatoes. I shudder at brown rice and organ meats, but have adequate amount of fish and grains in my weekly diet. I felt that I must ensure that I continued to include sufficient selenium rich foods in my diet as it appeared so necessary for good health.

Calcium I have always associated with bones and teeth but it is also important for the blood cholesterol levels and bloodclotting and most important for me was finding that heartbeat control, muscle and nerve functioning were also dependent on the presence of calcium. The richest natural sources were to be found in cheese, fish, nuts, root vegetables, eggs, milk, molasses, bread and yoghurt. I felt confident that I ate sufficient of this mineral in my normal diet but to add just a little extra was easily done and as my heart obviously needed some help then I could certainly give it in a dietary capacity.

After considerable retrospective reflection I was confident that I had learned all that I could about Wolff-Parkinson-White syndrome and accepted the probable causes of it and more important how I could help myself by re-balancing my diet. I was now confident that I could cope and in time win – nothing was going to stop me becoming the epitome of complete fitness. As soon as I took positive steps to help myself I was immediately uplifted and I never worried – such a negative pessimistic attitude was not part of my life in any way and never would be. What I did accept was that often I was the complete antithesis of relaxation and I now needed to concentrate on this, as I readily admitted that I still found this difficult. Stress must be eradicated before it eradicated me and after all the years of hard work and educating myself to lift my life on to the highest plateau of well-being, every part of me must unite in an amalgam of perfection. Stress had to go.

19

LESLEY

A Long time ago I had occasionally visited our local Cancer Support Group and they continued to send me their monthly newsletter. On glancing through this I saw that a class for meditation was held by a Lesley Barnes. As I knew that the more relaxed I could be would greatly benefit my heart and as I always felt better at such times I decided to arrange a visit. The first time that I spoke to her I was immediately aware of the rich timbre of her voice and waited impatiently for our first meeting.

After many aborted arrangements the evening of our meeting finally arrived, but with rain so torrential that I was filled with dismay, and when the telephone rang and it was Lesley to enquire "Did I want to cancel the evening?" I was so disappointed she said that she was quite happy to come in the rain if I wanted her to. I was relieved and told her that weather never put me off so we braved the monsoon deluge that made rivers and lakes of the road and arrived completely drenched but delighted to meet after so long. That was to be the beginning of a special relationship where over the months Lesley became a mixture of friend, twin soul and confident and taught me how to achieve a new and mystical dimension to my life. She was a laughing sonsy girl from Glasgow similar in age to myself, with a cloud of thick dark hair and a bright smile. From our first meeting I felt happy to be near her and the open face and clarity of vision that emanated from her person encouraged me to accept the welcomed spontaneity that she gave. She had had many heartaches during her life and lived in many places before settling quite close to where I had spent my childhood. She appeared so well and contented and full of energy I could hardly believe that she had suffered from multiple sclerosis for over twenty years and had had numerous operations and treatments for three different types of cancer. She seemed incapable of bearing a grudge against the many misfortunes life had dealt her. Over the ensuing weeks we learned about each other becoming friends, and in her company she taught me a plane of relaxation that I had not known. Bodily I could relax and this was a great help as Lesley showed me her individual way to relax my mind.

Normally all of my self help had been totally alone in a quiet house and here we had a room in the middle of our town and were in close proximity in its dimly lit smallness and I was acutely conscious of her presence. We began to meet once a week and I feel that nineteen ninety was the year of Lesley's influence as she was the first person in many years whom I felt had something important to offer me, without at first realising what it was. She had the elusive quality of radiating warmth, as if she were standing in a shaft of sunlight that drew me forward until I was enveloped in its security. Always she was kind and had that gift of being interested in other people, not burdening me with her problems but giving her whole attention to me until we shared that unique indefinable specialness. Over a period of time we only had to look at each other to know how we felt – whether the previous week had been fraught with frustrations or whether we were both on a high because we had felt well and had enjoyed ourselves. Lesley gave a lot to me and I like to think that I contributed something as she told me that she looked forward to our meeting with pleasurable anticipation. We would be eager to shut ourselves away from the happy chatter of the other members of the Group and go into our world of precious stolen time and share confidences like good friends can.

Jamie, so quiet, without confidence and tongue tied on meeting people for the first time took an immediate liking to Lesley. She found time to practise French with him and to improve his accent. I was amazed to see him drawn to her and joining in her making a fun time of his homework. Later he always referred to her as a "smiley" person and this was a shrewd and true remark. I never underestimate the intuitiveness of young people who can so often instinctively know the people who will never hurt them and can be confided in and trusted. His description of her was apt as her whole being was of happiness and she wanted to encompass everyone. She had a marvellous presence that you felt your soul uplifted by just being near her, Jamie was right; everyone became smiley when with Lesley.

When we were together and in accord, Lesley would play her cassette tape of mellow water music. Quietly it would fill the dimly lit room as we sat in harmony together. I would close my eyes and untense my body and breathe evenly and gently as Lesley began to speak in her sonorous voice that was music in itself as she transported us to the gentle make-believe world that she invented for us of green pastureland, mighty proud trees shrouding a wide cloudless sky and lazy stream. Already I was well aware of the pleasures to be gained from natural surroundings, but Lesley in her poetry took us both to new heights of awareness. We would walk barefoot in a green meadow feeling the earth's goodness and strength penetrate the soles of our feet, surrounded by nature's song. We would pause and gaze at a copper beech tree with the rustle of summer turning its dense foliage into a mirage of music of the sea and become encircled by glistening sound beneath an azure sky as the sunlight dappled through the leaves onto our upturned faces. We would feel the firm rough bark of the tree and take strength from its solidity and continue towards the sound of water by an old wooden bridge, aware of the lush green grass cool against our bare legs. We would walk on the uneven planks and gaze down at the sparkling clear water as it wended its way to fulfilment and we would sit on the bank and touch a yellow buttercup growing there; admire its dainty bell and see the golden dust on our fingers from its centre, never to be picked, just touched lightly as it grew to cast a small shadow on the water. Our bare toes would touch the water that was warm and inviting, so clear that the irregularity of the stones could clearly be seen with tufts of moss gracefully moving in a gentle current. We would enter the water and feel it close over us as we lay down, it soothed our bodies and trailed our hair as we were wafted along the enchanted waters of the hesitant elysian stream, the sun warming our upturned faces and reeds clinging to our outstretched arms before reluctantly letting us pass on our magical way. The creamy cadences of Lesley's voice softened into almost a whisper as the rhythmic movement of our bodies in the steam became relaxed as we floated as if into a space of pure harmony deep in the colours of light and drew in deeply of the peace and tranquillity of blissful meditation, when the body and soul soar to the heights of our utopia. We could feel our bodies move to higher planes, suspended in a vastness of radiant rich light that came ever closer until it invaded our beings and filled us with new life full of force but extreme gentleness. It would recede only to come closer again with its soft purity until we were enveloped in a rosy blush of universal goodness where we seemed to be actually outside our bodies and viewing them from silken shadows as they floated on a sea of glistening clarity. Our minds and bodies found complete freedom satiated in perfection that could not be tarnished but glowed protectingly around and into us. There was nothing mythical in our transcending beyond our former limits of experience and knowledge but the mystical and tangible realisation that we were experiencing an immediate intuition, an almost spiritual insight which was raising us higher than we could ever have contemplated. It was a rare inner light of rapture that was wholly of goodness. We would effortlessly stay suspended in infinity until, gently Lesley would bring us into the calm waters on the verge of the stream where we would descend lightly in our dream state. The water flowed from us leaving us dry and immune to all mediocrity and totally at peace. Gradually we became aware of the daily sounds around us as reluctantly we opened our eyes and left our private world until another time, secure in the knowledge that it was always there beckoning us invitingly to renew the ability that we had of regaining tranquillity.

Lesley had recorded her own words on a cassette "The Rainbow Dove" and she gave me a copy to use when at home. I could close my eyes and her richly resonant voice was reassuringly with me but in no wise was it like the reality. Over the months I learned from reading many books the depths and advantages of meditation. The whole purpose of meditation is inner happiness and peace and it has, like everything else, to be learned. The younger and untried you are the easier it is as life usually tends to obscure the natural tendencies of the body and mind and these foreign feelings have to be eliminated and replaced by the simple qualities that make for a person filled with love and understanding. Meditation is a natural function that we are practising in all the good in our daily lives and all this needs is to be recognised and developed and expanded until life's hurts can hardly touch us. Relaxing the mind and body helps educate the nervous system and feeds the brain until you can feel it expanding and thirsting for knowledge. Once the mind and body realise that you want to fill them with all that is pure, they will become eager and responsive as they want no banalities but all powerful inspiration, love and stimulation to find all that we need which is inside our beings but with patience has to be brought out and then used daily for total fulfilment of everyone's potentiality.

To help encompass meditation start in a small way and do everything that you do with complete concentration and with the best of your ability so that on its completion you will know satisfaction. Be patient, disassociate yourself from all distractions of loud discordant noise. Learn from others, but only believe and trust in that which you have experienced and therefore know to be true. I have learned automatically to recognise almost instantly the people from whom I can gain and they have taught me often without realising it. Be receptive to all that others can offer you and know also the people who should be avoided as this new awareness of life will not tolerate being sullied. Find your own way to total physical and mental relaxation when you will be ready to meditate and reap the high reward of mind and body being attuned. Give yourself time to think; it is the source of power and the prelude to true understanding, and always remember, there is no-one for whom no stars shine.

20

NATURAL HEALING

Spiritual Healing

Lesley knew that I was always interested in new ways to improve my life and one day she asked had I ever had any healing? Vaguely I recalled when on holiday in Criccieth my neighbour Gabrielle invited me to her home where I met her friend Mavis who she said was a Healer and had greatly helped her as she had been plagued with back problems for the many years that I had known her. Gabrielle was a devout Irish Catholic and incredibly beautiful with deep blue eyes in a perfect face with masses of blonde hair and a wonderful figure. Her lilting accent always seemed to me rather incongruous in the very Welsh Criccieth and caused me to smile on hearing her on our first visit of the year. With four children and a block of holiday flats to look after she still looked perfectly groomed, poised and elegant. I have never seen her look less than immaculate and she is the sort of person film stars are made of. In spite of her physical perfections she has always been content to be at home and a devoted wife and mother. She is so sincere that when she encouraged me to talk to Mavis I agreed. Mavis was a quiet person who initially seemed overshadowed by Gabrielle's exuberance, but as I talked to her I found her kindly. She said that she would like to help and placed her hands on me. I do not feel that I gave her a great deal of attention as there were a number of us in the room and Gabrielle as usual was full of fun and laughter, but I did feel a warmth emanate from Mavis to me. Afterwards Gabrielle said I seemed more relaxed and she was right. For all her gaiety she was a shrewd person. I remembered this meeting as Lesley told me that there were two healers who came to the group most weeks, Dennis and Rhona. She suggested that I arrange to see Dennis and I agreed. This was a field about which I knew nothing and was intrigued to learn what it entailed. Over many months now I had realised that Lesley was a special sort of person and if she thought that healing would help me then I would certainly accept openly any assistance that it could give me.

As soon as Lesley introduced me to Dennis I realised that I had met him at one of the social meetings of the Group sometime before, but not known that he was a healer. He was an impressive figure, tall and well made, and I recalled the first time that I had met him. I had immediately felt a power within him as he held my hand and had noticed how gentle he was in spite of his large person. Even then as I had looked at him I had felt the presence of goodness that he exuded.

My meetings with Lesley became important to me as the weeks continued and as our time together clashed with the time that Dennis was at the Group, for a long time I hardly saw him at all. Early in November 1990 Lesley was too unwell for our weekly meeting, so I suggested that maybe I take the opportunity of seeing Dennis. She agreed that this was a good idea and I contacted Dennis who fortunately was at the Group that evening. It was with some curiosity that I went with him to one of the rooms set aside for special counselling and I told him that I had no idea what he would do, but as Lesley had recommended that he could help me I was in no doubt that he would be able to do so.

We sat quietly in the cosy dimly lit room which invited confidences and he said that I had nothing to be afraid of. We would share a short time of relaxation and prayers together when he would sit beside me. He explained that he had great faith in our Creator who would decide how I would be helped. Dennis asked if I had any particular physical pains that bothered me most and I said that my heart condition still frightened me during the times when I felt ill but for the most part I had learned how to cope with it. He understood how I felt and I leaned back in the comfortable chair and closed my eyes as he said just relax with him. The physical relaxation that I had learned so long ago I now did automatically and felt a warmth as I went into the now familiar limbo state, but being fully aware of what was going on. Dennis put his hands close to me, just barely touching my hair and I felt the waves of warmth flowing into my body. He continued to sit by me and the whole room seemed full of his serenity. I was aware vaguely of the talking and laughter in the social room up above, but felt quite unaffected by it, being content to be cocooned in this new way to help myself. Of course I feel that my attitude of complete optimism in accepting the people who can help me and giving myself into their hands with trust is the best way to benefit from this spiritual help and I knew that further meetings with Dennis would help me in a way that no-one else had. He said that he could tell that I had pain in my lower back and abdomen which was true but he had no way of knowing that. He made a number of comments that confirmed my initial feelings that this person had great insight to others and that his kind eyes belied the depth of intensity within him. I knew that in him I had found another person who would assist me. The intrinsic goodness of Dennis had the power to give aid by my just talking to him anywhere at any time. I learned that a healer is always "switched on" and in a crowded room over many months I have felt a peace engulfing me and on turning have seen Dennis smile reassuringly. I feel protected when he is near me.

Relaxation

In my pursuit to explore all avenues to achieve total relaxation I joined Yvonne's class at our Support Group. As always the atmosphere was happy and welcoming and Yvonne a kind quietly spoken person. I told her that I felt better just being with her and was not surprised when she told me that she used to be a healer. She said that she had never trained as a counsellor as she felt that her gift came from God and she was right. Goodness and a genuine desire to help other people cannot be taught. It has to come from inside and if it is there you will instinctively know how to use these gifts. I had already appreciated this from time spent with Dennis.

We sat comfortably as Yvonne initially asked us to participate in a few gentle exercises; or, if we were unable, just to sit quietly and join in when we wished. She then asked us to relax our forehead, neck and head with gentle massage. She showed us how to breathe deeply and evenly but without any force. It is impossible to remain tense when you have learned to breath correctly. She said that we should find time every day to relax the body, mind and spirit. She asked us to relax our toes, then feel the warmth of the relaxation continue into our ankles, calves then thighs, up into our hips and body. We relaxed our fingers that rested in our laps, feeling the relaxation creeping into our hands, our wrists and the whole of our arms. She said to let go the worries and burdens from our shoulders and feel the tension easing in our neck as the relaxation continued, gently smoothing away the worry lines on our brow and feeling the eyes relax and if the lids were tightly closed then releasing them a little. Yvonne asked us to feel the cheeks relax and unclench the teeth and let the tongue relax in the mouth. The whole body was now relaxed and one felt good.

Yvonne asked if we had heard of the existence of the electromagnetic energy field surrounding the body called the aura – I had to admit that I hadn't. She explained that this is an area of energy which surrounded every living thing, vegetables, flowers, trees, animals and humans. It could extend for miles on highly evolved souls and counsellors and healers usually had strong auras and this made them acutely receptive to other peoples problems and they could often sense if they were unwell just by looking at them. The aura contains our thoughts both positive and negative and all our thoughts and actions are recorded in it. It was important that we cleanse the aura because all illness starts there. We can pick up other peoples negativity as well as our own, so it was important to protect oneself against this. I found this fascinating as I certainly found that when I was with miserable and pessimistic people I could feel myself sinking mentally and spiritually and on leaving them felt low. Conversely being with bright positive fun people had the opposite effect and if I felt a little down on meeting them I could feel myself becoming lifted in their presence and in a short time felt so much better and on leaving them could be quite elated. When we receive an injury or become ill this energy field is disturbed and out of balance. Or, if the aura itself is out of balance, then physical symptoms will begin to manifest in time. I had found out myself that good thinking would help my health and bad thinking would be negative.

She asked us to imagine drawing in light through the top of the head, first from close to the body and then from further away; repeating this made you feel surrounded by a warm glow that you were able to draw into your body. She then asked us to draw in the earth's energy up through the feet and right through the body and this repeated makes you feel much stronger.

We then relaxed quietly with eyes closed as she played gentle music with natural bird sounds with which I was immediately wafted into the vastness of a countryside alive with natures song, as Yvonne's soft yet authorative voice took us along a country lane full of the joy of life on a summer day. We would walk up to a white gate over which could be glimpsed a meadow and we would pause as Yvonne asked us to take from our shoulders the burdens and worries of life that we had and put them down at the side of the lane. It was a great relief to do this and immediately I felt my spirits rise as I went to the gate and opened it and entered a meadow with a floor covered with the colours of wild flowers. The inquisitive hedgrow fronds tickled my cheek as they lightly brushed my face as I hesitated before walking softly over the flowers, so light and free that no head was crushed and made my way to a bridge over a stream of crystal clear chattering water and crossed it and continued to the foot of a high mountain. With Yvonne leading us we spiritually climbed the heights – more floating than climbing, passing grazing sheep on our way and taking pleasure of a light breeze and appreciating the colours of the wild flowers and trees that we passed. Effortlessly we reached the top and lay in the grass warmed by the sun that entered our bodies as we lay at peace. We rested for a while in tune with all that was good before descending full of contentment as we crossed the bridge and the enchanted meadow and out into the lane. We paused briefly by our heavy burdens and left them where they had been placed and continued back into the world again. This was a particular favourite picture story of mine and Yvonne had many, all so different but all equally relaxing and a pleasure to participate in. For a while we would just sit quietly together with closed eyes until the sounds of everyday life invaded our minds and I stretched and felt good as I joined in the general talk of our happy and now relaxed group. I always felt refreshed after our weekly class and looked forward to our meetings. I learned a great deal from Yvonne and was grateful to her in always being ready to help me at any time that she could. She truly is a natural healer.

If anyone doubts the benefits obtained from relaxation I saw at first hand the power of good that it can do. Recently whilst waiting for Yvonne to begin our class an anxious young man came into the room with his wife. She was completely distraught,in tears and her whole body shaking uncontrollably. Yvonne, who is one of the most sympathetic and compassionate people that you would wish to meet, immediately tried to comfort her and on calming her a little suggested that she join in the waiting class. I think that it was with reluctance that she agreed and sat rigidly on the edge of one of the settees. With wide eyes she watched Yvonne and followed her lead until gradually she became more calm. By the end of the class she was entirely in control of herself and her tears had given way to a smile as she made ready to leave. I think it helped her knowing that most of us in the room had at some time felt exactly as she had and we all gave her our quiet support in her distress. If ever I needed proof of the power of natural healing surely this was it.

Having been made aware of the existence of the aura and its importance by Yvonne, I decided to read all I could about it as I had decided long ago that however unusual and obscure something seemed to me initially, if it was natural and beneficial to health then it would be fitted into my lifestyle.

A form of photography pioneered by Semyon Kirlian in Russia in 1939 has put the whole subject of auras on a more scientific basis. Kirlian photography captures the interaction between the electro-magnetic energy and a high-voltage electrical field. This diagnosis has been used extensively in the Eastern Block; during the 1970s, Rumania alone had fourteen thousand state-aided scientists developing the idea for political and medical use. Despite having been available in Britain for over fifteen years, Kirlian photography is still relatively unknown. Kirlian consultants say that they can give a 'snapshot' of your physical and mental health. Basic personality traits are constant but changes in fatigue and stress levels can be seen within a day. The process involved standing in a darkened room for twelve seconds with hands on a sheet of photographic paper placed on a plain white box. The aura emerged as black blobs and a vague fuzzy outline of parts of the hands. To me aura pictures are nothing like any ordinary photographs, but have an incandescent beauty with light flashes reminiscent of the most brightly coloured fireworks with the brilliant glow of stars and all in technicolour.

"Feeling blue" being "green with envy" or in "black despair" may be more than just everyday phrases. Psychics claim that we all go round showing our true colours. The way we feel is, they say, reflected in our auras – bands of coloured light that surround us and that only specially gifted people can see under normal circumstances. Experts say that Kirlian photography enables you to see a picture of the life-force itself, raw energy fizzing out from anything that lives – humans, animals, leaves, flowers, even crystals and minerals. Healthy creatures give off the most impressive light shows. Sick or unhappy ones have unhappy or dull auras, sometimes even with holes! If you are depressed, it will dwindle almost to nothing. Huge bursts of light show spiritual energy as well as physical well-being. Healers, for example, give off great flashes when preparing to heal. A coin shows up as a living thing. This comes from the energy from it being handled by so many people who have left their mark on it. Fruit picked straight off the tree shows the biggest Kirlian flare. Fruit kept in a bowl for a week registers almost dead. A Kirlian photograph of a leaf will show its faint outline left behind; maybe connected with the phantom limb phenomenon, where an amputated leg or arm still hurts.

The photographs have colour codes, Grey: lacking in energy, low in health and perhaps feeling depressed. Blue: calm, serene and religiously inclined, maybe lacking in warmth. Violet/Indigo: highly evolved spiritually and possibly out of touch with reality. Yellow: plenty of energy and optimism, but lacking spiritually. Orange: vital and sunny but not always sympathetic to others. Red: fiery and a good leader. The aura pictures are some of the most incredibly beautiful in their mystery that I have ever seen and I truly believe that they depict life, as they themselves are bright as lightning and sharp as a staccato beat. If I am ever fortunate enough to have the opportunity of participating in Kirlian photography I shall accept immediately, eager to learn of its findings of me.

Reflexology

Reflexology is the art of healing through foot massage. It is an approach to the care of the entire body which uses the feet to stimulate healing. It works on the energy fields in the body, balancing the flow of energy. It improves the blood supply to areas and seems to be able to reduce nervous tension in different parts of the body, giving a relaxing effect. Reflexology, or reflex zone therapy of the feet, has linked the feet to each organ in the body, creating a map to read and assess the health of the patient. Each part of us is linked to our feet by an invisible thread via which weakness and disease can be discerned and eventually eradicated by therapeutic massage. It has its roots in ancient folk medicine – the ancient Chinese, Egyptians and Red Indian tribes used foot massage as a form of healing. The concept of the body's reflexes and using them for therapeutic purposes has also been around for centuries – the ancient Chinese developed the technique of acupressure, the basis of which lies in the knowledge of reflex zones and connections between different parts of the body.

At the beginning of this century Dr. Fitzgerald, an American Ear, Nose and Throat expert, noticed that making minute surgical incisions on some of his patients caused different reactions in different individuals – thus rediscovering the concept that pressure points on the body have reflective connections in other areas. Dr. Fitzgerald created his own version of acupressure points by dividing the body into ten zones, running from the top of the head to the tips of the toes. His body zones comprised two series of five longitudinal zones, each of which finished in a corresponding finger or toe. The theory was that everything occurring in a specific zone of the body affects and is influenced by the organs and other parts of the body in that zone. All the reflex zones on the feet are massaged in an attempt to discover weak or diseased parts of the body. If a particular reflex zone was painful during massage, the related area of the body was likely to be functioning below par. The self-healing ability of the body reacted to the healing stimulus. Reflexology began to spread both among the American general public and in medical circles. Eunice Ingham, a young masseuse, introduced a special grip technique in the action of the thumb on the foot and developed a more intricate zone system with areas pinpointed on toes, sole and ankle of each foot. This idea spread, and it was introduced by Doreen Bayly into England in the 1960s and she set up the Bayly School of Reflexology in 1978. Hanna Marquardt, who like Doreen Bayly was influenced by Eunice Ingham, developed the reflex zone concept, introducing various zones which were previously unknown or uncertain and consequently the International School of Reflex Zone Therapy of the Feet grew up, which now has branches all over the world.

Imagine my interest when I met Jean, a reflexologist who helped people at our Group, who was more than willing to add me to her long waiting list. Many of the members of our Group told me how they had benefited from her treatment and how relaxing the therapy was. As relaxation was a top priority with me I was more than eager to learn from her the secrets of this previously unknown therapy. I had noticed Jean before without realising who she was. She was incredibly quick and slim with loose curly hair and large bright eyes in a kitten face. Of all the people at the Group I always thought of her as the most glamourous as she was so chic with the air of a Parisienne.

I went with Jean to her reflexology room which she had decorated and furnished herself. It was warm and her personal touches gave a prelude to relaxation. I was made comfortable in a large lounger as I found this preferable to her table. It was serene and quiet with only soft music playing as my first session started with Jean lightly dusting my right foot with talc before examining it closely. She started with my toes before passing to the sole of my foot, seeming to me to be tracing hidden lines over my foot. Most of the time it was just so pleasant to feel her firm but gentle touch, but occasionally her fingers would draw a line and it was as if a lighted fuse was running along my foot, and I could almost hear the crackle, that I could certainly feel like electric shocks, but it was not unpleasant. She massaged my ankle and the top of my foot, sometimes seeming to pull it gently and occasionally to make sweeping movements from my foot to my lower leg. Gradually I sank further into the chair, only being aware of Jean's touch of rhythmic movements, until she transferred to my left foot. An hour went by before I was reluctantly brought back to reality feeling pleasantly tired. I had not been asleep, but in a half world of semi-state, blissfully free of bodily trappings as I floated in euphoric ecstacy. My feet seemed to be alive and "working" and this glow lasted a number of hours. It was as if they had been stimulated into life after being dormant. Jean told me that my muscle tone was poor and that reflexology would help this. She demonstrated what she meant by holding my foot up which dropped limply when she loosed it. If I were in better condition this would not happen. She also volunteered that generally I was not robust and I had to agree with her. She asked whether I suffered with backache and I told her that I had intermittently since the birth of Jamie but how I improved this with my back support chair and careful symmetrical movements. When I told her that I always had a daily walk she said that this was good and would also help my muscle tone.

I explained to Jean my need to relax to help my heart condition and on answering her enquiry as to the nature of it, I was surprised that she knew of it and actually knew someone else who had my syndrome. She quickly told me that she could not cure this and I said I hardly expected her to, just to help me generally and I would continue to cope with the syndrome myself. She was confident that she could help me and suggested that to help myself I give up ten minutes a day to listen to music and relax, not just to fit it in sometimes or around a busy day but to set a time for myself daily, preferably the same time each day and to devote it to myself. Jean was a shrewd person and I felt she could understand exactly the sort of person that I was and the ease with which she diagnosed my problems I would have found uncanny if it had not been for the enormous respect that I now had for all natural healers. I never question how they do it, how they seem to look into one's soul and formulate an accurate picture of one's life and difficulties. It is enough to me that they do it. All therapists seemed to have a good rapport with their patients, probably founded on their genuine interest in helping with their own special gift and of course in giving that priceless commodity – their time. All of these healers were so different in their chosen fields and yet all in harmony in their wish to give of themselves to help in their own soothing miraculous way. To me they complemented each other perfectly. I could not fail to be helped with so much rich advice available and willingly given to me. I promised Jean that I would find time for myself and she said that I must learn to give myself time – and her parting words were that I must learn to love myself.

Chromotherapy

Chromotherapy or colour healing has been in use since ancient times. The Greeks and Egyptians knew of its power and the influence of colour is shown in the great Egyptian temples, such as Karnak and Thebes, where there were colour halls where research into the use of colour and colour healing was practised.

In more recent times colour therapy has been in use for approximately ten years and was another fascinating world for me and introduced by Marilyn, a piquant-faced girl with English rose colouring. She explained that the spine was used for diagnosis, as all major systems were attached to the spine. This was split into four sections, the physical, metabolic, emotional and mental, and these had their own corresponding colours. Marilyn explained that light was energy and therefore the sun had great energy. When light is broken it breaks into different colours and each colour has a different energy wavelength. Each wavelength had certain qualities which can be used to benefit our health. Colour Therapy worked first on the aura with which I now felt familiar and then the physical body. We all have an aura around us consisting of energy bands of colours of the spectrum. When the body's energies become unbalanced colours help to restore it. They were more than hues and had a power of healing – Red for energy – which also makes us feel warm, Orange for joy, Yellow for detachment, Green for balance, Turquoise for purity, Blue for calmness and relaxation, which also makes us feel cold,

Violet for respect and Magenta to help let go. The aura contained many colours, the paler and more refined the aura and colour the more spiritual the person. Bright colours like red denoted vibrant positive people. This reminded me of all that Yvonne had previously explained to me. I did feel that all these natural healers overlapped each other in a complementary way enabling me to obtain the best out of them all without any jarring notes.

As I explained my great wish to relax, Marilyn suggested that blue would be a beneficial colour for me, as this was most relaxing – in fact she volunteered that she had a "Blue" room at home. This could be helped by using a blue light bulb and wearing blue clothing. I did know this to be true as over many years I had felt the calming influence of a room at my mother's home which was predominately blue – which was her favourite colour with rich silk curtains and multi-blue coloured wool carpet. I only had to walk into the room and stand for a few moments to feel its cool calmness enveloping me.

I sat with Marilyn in one of our quiet rooms while she asked me a few brief questions about myself. She lit a candle and she said that she found this helps stillness and is calming and was also used as protection from other people's energies. She gave me a therapy chart on which was drawn the spine. On the reverse side I drew a line along the outline of the spine and then added my name along it. From this Marilyn proceeded to colour my chart, dowsing with her fingers as she did so. I sat and watched as she added brightness to the paper, content that my life would never be of linear design, but with all this new found knowledge I would extend to the farthest periphery. To my curious gaze it just looked like a growing mass of colour, but to her it told an amazingly accurate story of myself. She could tell that I was tense and that this could have enamated as far back as childhood fears. I said that I had attended a strict primary school by today's standards and had not been happy. Not that I ever wanted to break the rules but that I had found the forbidding severe nature of the teachers not easy to accept and those early years had not been a fun time as I feel early learning should be. She said that I had to look into these fears and understand and accept them and then learn to put them behind me forever and this would help me be more relaxed. She also asked me whether I enjoyed my food as this had showed up as a problem area. This seemed an amazing question as I loved every mouthful that I ate and I said that I certainly did. When I explained that I was under a great deal of stress she said that this was showing upon the spinal picture as a lack of joy, because problems were also upsetting my bodily balance. I knew that food eaten at times of stress was less beneficial than it should be, but unfortunately it was not always possible to eliminate it. I explained to her that I coped with it now far better than I used to.

Marilyn asked me to take off my outer clothes and put on a loose white cotton garment and lie on the table. She then placed over me a cloth of natural fabric of turquoise which the spine chart had shown was needed. She remarked that I had chosen for that day to wear a turquoise jumper which had been the right decision and I said I always did as my body directed and I just knew that this was the right colour for me to wear. She dimmed the room and played soft music before scanning my body with her hands – close, but not touching me. After a while she changed the cloth covering me to a red one which she said would give energy and help my low blood pressure. She also said that a predominately red room would give energy, but would be too much to be in for long. She then repeated the covering of turquoise before scanning my body for the last time. This time she gently but firmly held my head and then touched my hands and fingers to take away any negative energies. Scanning the body with her hands enabled her to check where there were any blockages and she could tell that the area of my heart was heavy and that a course of therapy would help. By this time I felt relaxed and totally at ease as I lay quietly listening to the music and appreciating just how much these people who understood natural medicine could help. My heart was now beating so normally that it was hardly discernable and this more than anything told me that Marilyn was another gem that I had had the good fortune to meet. She told me that she was not a trained counsellor but that colour therapy was treating the spiritual as well as the physical body, and I recognised in her this warm sympathetic understanding of other people that was apparent in healers. When I asked whether she found therapy draining for her she said that it was sometimes and I could understand this as she gave so much of herself.

I was interested when she said that great stress could lead to lack of magnesium and that magnesium helped the electrical impulses in the heart to travel correctly. This again confirmed what I had long thought, that stress was my greatest enemy in correcting my heart rhythm. I checked and confirmed that magnesium was necessary for the normal working of the heart and with energy production. Richest food sources were wheat bran, green vegetables – the greener the better, the magnesium being present in the chlorophyll, whole grains, nuts, seafood, lentils, soya beans and brown rice. Tap water in hard water areas was also an important source. It was easy for me to have just a little extra of the necessary foods but not so easy to dismiss stress, but I was going to with the help of Marilyn.

Marilyn suggested that I try painting to help express myself through creativity. Initially I could try drawing – something that I cared for, maybe a bird visiting my garden. Immediately I thought of the abundance of wildlife liberally on my doorstep. My exquisite fox family of responsible parents and adorable inquisitive young would make enchanting subjects. So too would the dumpy wood pigeons forever on my lawns and the effortless grace of naughty squirrels as they flew between the trees stealing my raspberries and apples cried out to be captured on canvas. Small but in no way insignificant were my mouse residents of the garden shed, scurrying plump bundles of brown fur that would give enchanting life to a pastoral scene. Painting the beauty of a single flower could also express my love of nature. I pondered on Marilyn's words of encouragement as I had a high regard for her and realised that these ideas were none that I doubt I would have ever thought of and up until now no-one else had suggested painting. For many years now I had appreciated the works of the great masters so why shouldn't I try to make a masterpiece of my own? An idyllic summer country setting of green fields and tall trees and maybe a stream or lazy river meandering its dreamy way to the sea were my favourite places to be at every opportunity. It would be so easy to take a pad of empty pages and pencils and then to take a few tentative strokes to make a picture. Whatever my choice, I knew that Marilyn was right when she said that this would help, just as long as I painted or drew with love for my subject. Brian was no artist but Jamie certainly was and amongst his many talents was an aptitude for artistic creativity. Marilyn's idea would be a new way for us to spend a precious day out and what fun we would have in making our personal mementoes.

Colour coding was another dimension of colour therapy that Marilyn offered to do for me. This analysis would be based on my natural colouring of hair, eyes and skin. She invited me to sit in front of a large mirror which I found rather daunting as I can say with honesty that I never sit in this way normally. She wrapped a neutral coloured cape around my shoulders and then placed beside me a large pile of coloured pieces of cloth of all imaginable shades. She explained that from these she would select the colours most suited to me – not only for their appearance but also they could be worn for their health-giving properties when needed. Before starting she said that although my hair was so dark and also my eyes, there was a clarity and brightness in them too and that my skin was olive toned. The colours which would make me at my most attractive were the ones which would harmonise with my natural dark tones and clear brightness – but not too bright! The idea of being colour analysed was to help people see how good they could look, which would boost their morale, giving them confidence and a self esteem which could literally transform people in the best possible way. It was so easy to forget or not to realise how good you could look, having lost or not known your self worth.

Marilyn commenced by taking a coloured cloth from the top of the pile and placing it across my shoulder. At first all the colours seemed attractive to me, but I soon realised that not all suited me. What at first seemed a gorgeous brilliance of varied colour soon established a pattern and it emerged even to my untrained eye that colours of a deep hue and a definite brightness, without overshadowing me, were most suitable. Marilyn explained that all the colour tones that she used were split into types, these being bright, light, dark, deep, cool, warm and muted and that she categorised me as being dark and bright. Also some colours looked good against my skin whilst others were preferable away from my face, as could be worn in a jacket or suit. I became more intrigued with her unusual expertise as she progressed, until we were both immersed in her colourful world. What was obvious from the onset was how uplifting and happy all of this therapy was and you just had to feel better with so much colour to cheer you.

Marilyn sifted through the colours, some to be discarded and some to be placed aside as being complementary to me. I was disappointed that one of my favourite colours, yellow, made me look sallow and accentuated my olive skin that in no way enhanced it. I asked Marilyn whether she thought the large amount of carrots that I consumed were the cause of my skin colour. She thought it could accentuate it but that it was more likely to be my own personal body makeup.

Colours that looked particularly good and made me "come alive" were rich emerald green and deep emerald/turquoise and a merge of blue and green that held a touch of aquamarine. I was so pleased that my favourite colour suited me so well as I could never imagine myself without verdant shades in my wardrobe. I was surprised that a warm purple looked advantageous against my skin as I had always thought this too sombre for me, but Marilyn cleverly showed me with her varieties of the same colour that a shade of difference was all that was needed to find a head turning choice. Of these colours which came under the heading of dark/bright the deep rose was my favourite. Its depth of colour made a glow of my face and I decided that this was a colour that I would want to wear. Of the deep colours pine and forest green were chosen and a blue-red reminiscent of a fresh raspberry. A clear pillar box red that was a vibrant shade and bright burgundy were on my plus pile and I was gratified that a golden yellow suited me. The golden tone tempered the yellow and it was exactly right for me. Of the dark/muted list I could wear a dark tomato red and autumn rust were chosen and would warm a cold winter day for the future, brightened up with gold jewellery. It was interesting that although we now had a large pile of cloths of suitable colours I had to learn which were best close to my face to obtain maximum effect from them. All of these lessons were a delight to learn with such an able and happy teacher.

Oyster white, grey beige, light true grey, medium true grey, soft white, rose beige, charcoal grey, navy and dark chocolate brown could be used as my neutrals and were suitable for coat, jacket and skirt colours and of course trousers that were a vital part of my wardrobe for comfort and warmth. What I found incredible was that how attractive black looked on me particularly when tempered with a touch of gold with a necklace or scarf and particularly with golden earrings.

Marilyn also showed me the advantage of good colour combinations. Medium blue/green and royal blue – medium violet and rose beige – these colours looked exciting together as did deep rose and warm purple. These were ideas that would never have entered my head and of course the most startling and dramatic was of black and clear gold. Two absorbing hours had passed and it had been a delight to spend them with Marilyn, not only to learn from her but to spend them in her friendly company.

Of course I did appreciate that over the years all of this knowledge would need to be updated as my hair inevitably became more grey and my skin lost any early bloom but with Marilyn to help I was confident that not only could I become better in health but I could become more attractive as well.

Having ascertained the colours most suited to me and combinations of colours, Marilyn said she now had to decide my body type, so that I purchased garments of the correct shape and type of material. I looked questioningly at her and she gave as an example a plump person wearing ideal colour combinations, but of horizontal stripes which would accentuate excess of weight; being slim this type of material would be ideal for me. I understood what she was saying and at her request stood straight and took the pole that she handed to me. It was the height of my body with a length of weighted string attached, rather like a "plumb line", and Marilyn said that this was the way that it was used as the pole would give my figure shape, and the difference between it and the hang of the string would give her the knowledge that she needed to decide the shape of the clothes that would best suit me. The idea was to show up my good points and hide my bad ones!

At Marilyn's direction I moved the pole into various positions around my body and turned about as she requested as she watched and built up a complete picture of my body shape. Basically I was defined as "balanced" without any glaringly obvious peculiarities. My body type was straight with tapered shoulders with my waist in the correct place. The pole also ascertained that my whole body length was equal to that of my whole leg length. All of this was fun to do and gave Marilyn all the knowledge that she needed to design a wardrobe just for me.

Marilyn thought that my "positive" points were my hair, face, neck and shoulders and that these should be accentuated.

The material generally for my clothes should be of average scale patterns, weight of fabric, line, detail and accessories. Necklines and collars should not be too low; otherwise most types with straight lines; 'V' and square neck were suitable.

Blouses and tops would suit me best with straight yokes. Details on clothes like shoulder epaulettes and bust pockets would detract from my slimness, as would belted tunics, sweatshirts, jumpers and long waistcoats. I was pleased that I already had a number of these items so that it appeared that my choice coincided with the expertise of Marilyn!

Skirts could be of a variety – tapered, circular, dirndl and those with a centre detail. Flared, box, stitched and knife pleats were suitable as were culottes.

Dress styles favoured were the double breasted coat dress, drop waisted, low pleats, chemise, shift and blouson.

Trouser legs could be quite varied with leg types of eased pleats, straight, baggy, wide-legged and jeans.

Jackets and coats would be double or single breasted – some with cut away bottom. The long tunic was favoured, edge to edge and car coat, and items with straight yokes.

Sleeves should be set in, kimono, dolman or bishop with detailed or padded shoulders and cuffed, either long or short.

Pockets were best just below the waist or breast level.

Accessories like belts should be narrow, and useful shoe shapes were pumps, flat, boots, slingback, walking and sandals and this choice greatly pleased me as foot care was a top priority with me and comfort a necessity.

Handbag shapes should be predominantly square or longer in width but never of a vertical design.

Jewellery should be chosen to give width so that square and angled would be best or a little chunky. Marilyn suggested using clip-on earrings as a scarf pin or cuff links and I thought these novel ideas.

As I was slim the idea was to create the illusion of me having a fuller figure with wool fabrics or anything giving a chunky cuddly appearance. I agreed with all of Marilyn's suggestions and not only had we spent many hours when she had been my teacher, they had been fun times as well and we had the added joy of finding that we had a lot in common.

To add the final touches to my new colour aware self Marilyn offered to make up my face to enhance it and accentuate my "good qualities" I was rather dubious about this as I informed her that I hadn't worn make-up for years. When she volunteered the information that none of her make-up had been tested on animals and that she would use it sparingly, I agreed.

I sat in front of the now familiar mirror. Marilyn placed the protective cover over my shoulders and I watched her delve into her case as she sought the items that she required. She was incredibly light as quicksilver with swift bird-like movements and her elfin face made disbelief of the fact that she was a grandmother to babies Katie, Jane and Rebecca Susan as she hardly appeared old enough to be out of school herself. She was full of common sense and had easily given me good advice which I brought into my everyday life, and for which I was grateful.

Deftly she bid me close my eyes as she gently brushed the lids with highlighter, a light cream powdered eyeshadow and then outlined my eyes with dark brown eye shadow. My lids then received more powder of a bronzy-brown colour and my eyes were completed with a touch of black mascara. I said that the only mascara that I had ever used had been the block type applied with a brush which to me was always reminiscent of cleaning shoes (the result was probably the same as in those days I was rather heavy handed). I think Marilyn thought my make-up style suited to the dark ages and as I looked at her efforts my eyes looked much brighter and larger. I was pleased, and interested to sit back and let her continue. She requested that I allow her to pluck my eyebrows into a more elegant line and to this I gave a firm No! I would not submit to any beauty treatment that necessitated such pain and besides, I was satisfied with my generously proportioned eyebrows and had never felt the urge to alter their shape. Whilst accepting that looking as attractive as possible did give a fillip to my ego I had never been particularly dissatisfied with my appearance and vanity was an empty sin that I could never be accused of.

She explained that she wanted to obtain a natural look and applied blusher on and slightly under my cheek bones which immediately gave my face a more positive appearance. My lips she coloured first with a brown lip liner and then filled them in with a darker bronze shade lipstick. Alternatively Marilyn felt that red or deep pink would have been equally suitable. She stood behind me and we both surveyed her work. I certainly looked different. My eyes so much larger and my teeth white against the glowing lip-gloss and the blusher giving my face a healthy slightly sun-tanned glow. We agreed the make-up was a great enhancer and as Marilyn commented, I looked more in the land of the living. She explained that she took into account the colour of my hair, skin and eyes and then decided what harmonised best with my own natural colouring. As a piece de resistance she clipped on shiny golden ear-rings that brought out amber tints in my eyes. As I had such a warm colouring I should always wear golden jewellery and not silver. As Marilyn had used the minimum amount of makeup, was the transformation due totally to her undisputed skill or had I a hitherto un-thought-of innate glamour?

With her sympathetic understanding of colour in so many guises Marilyn had taught me a great deal, not least that because I had no wish to be a fashion plate of the catwalk model variety, did not mean that I could not use colours in my everyday life to my advantage, and we agreed that asking Brian for a new outfit of the suggested colours most suited to me an excellent idea.

On returning home I was eager to await Jamie's reaction as he had never seen me in make-up. He took one look and said that it didn't look like "me" and told me to take it off. I found this amusing, but was not sure that I wanted to return to what he was used to – someone mainly to be found in the kitchen, totally unadorned.

We went for our usual walk in the park and met Judith, an attractive girl with naturally curly titian hair who always used make-up sparingly but expertly applied. I asked for her comments and she considered me enhanced by Marilyn's subtle applications and we agreed that I harmonised well with her large five year old dog Sam who had come up to me for the expected fuss that he always received. He was a glorious mixture of alsation, collie and retriever with a thick coat a rainbow of all the shades of autumn bronze. Judith declined my offer to accept him as my own as he so well matched my "new look". Many years ago when I became aware of the importance of correct posture my mind would see brief subliminal cuts of Sam as he effortlessly wended his way round the park. Incredibly large, and in spite of being a mongrel – of a Crufts winner variety – he was so light on his paws that he seemed to glide with supple floating movements, the whole of his body in perfect symmetry. I learned a lot from watching the rippling motion of his thick fur as he drifted by, even more accentuated by the excitable hops of his two house companions, Jack Russells, Jack and Jilly.

Returning home I was well satisfied with my hours spent with Marilyn, not only learning from her but enjoying her cheerful companionship as well.

Crystal Therapy

Since deciding that natural healing was to be the foundation of my fitness regime, when my attention was drawn to the benefits of Crystal Therapy I was eager to learn more of this. On being informed that the intriguingly named shop "Wyvern" was only a few miles from where I lived, I set out to locate it in my quest to learn how I could help myself in all diverse ways.

Hidden behind a busy high street I found "Wyvern", instantly recognisable by its unusual logo, so tucked away that I would never have discovered it without explicit directions. On entering the small shop I was instantly aware of stepping into an immaculately laid out room aglow with the lights of hundreds of stones. Always acutely sensitive to atmosphere I felt a peace descend on me as I shut the door on the unwanted noise outside. There were so many stones of endless variety of colour and texture, some set into exquisite jewellery, some as polished stones and some with heavier density in their natural state.

Lesley, who had been expecting me to call, welcomed me and gave me a brief outline of how her partner Chris and herself were endeavouring to provide a therapy with crystals which were physically recuperative, as well as healing the heart and mind. They had been interested in minerals for a number of years and after learning themselves decided to open a shop which they had had for nearly two years. They had also written a book on the subject and gave talks at meetings held regularly for interested persons. I thought them most enterprising people and felt that they could teach me a great deal.

First I asked about the name and Lesley explained that the Wyvern was a two-legged dragon with feet like an eagle. Dragons were an ancient earth symbol and Wyverns were the guardians of the universe, holding the cosmic energies in balance. Their logo depicted the wings of the black and white Wyverns, intertwined in space and revolving through time. The two Wyverns represent the opposing, yet complimentary, forces at work in nature, the balance of which maintains the ordered universe. The white, feather-winged Wyvern represented light, summer, the sun and the sky. The black, web-winged Wyvern represented dark, winter, the moon and the waters. The white and black Wyverns hold each other's tails in their mouths, and spin eternally through the seasons. All of this I found enthralling and listened intently to all that she could tell me.

I learned how Chris had used holistic therapies to gain and enjoy good health and with therapeutic use of crystals, minerals and gems had become aware of and understood the emotional basis of good health and well-being. This therapy was focused on emotional rather than physical problems and helps to rebalance vital energies which in turn contributes towards healing bodily ills.

Lesley further explained to me that crystals, minerals and gemstones are used therapeutically to promote healing and to develop self-awareness. Emotional distress associated with ill-health, disability, family problems, work difficulties and bereavement can be resolved with crystal healing. Each natural stone has a unique vibrational energy which harmonises with a particular emotional state, and is used to bring about a feeling of emotional well-being.

How you feel about yourself colours the way you live your life. Emotional conflict within yourself, or in your relationships with others, can give rise to many different feelings. For instance, you may suffer with your nerves, lose your enjoyment of life or worry a lot. All too often people live in fear, feel indignant, lack confidence, or become depressed. You may cease to love yourself, or perhaps feel you never have, and this can depress your immune system, and so lower your resistance to disease.

Crystal Therapy reduces accumulated stress, improves rest and relaxation, and releases energy to revitalise your life. It can help you to develop self-awareness and self-acceptance, so that you can find your direction in life and realise your full potential. It enhances feelings of strength and protection, improves motivation and increases your experience of fun and laughter in your life.

From the recesses of my mind I recalled visiting a shop "The Mineral Kingdom" in Abersoch and "The Fossil Shop" at Lyme Regis a decade ago where my eyes had briefly lit on this awareness of the powers of natural stones but I had not pursued it and realised that this was my loss which I was now fortunate enough to be able to rectify.

Lesley ascertained that different stones were beneficial for different emotions, but to a large extent each person needed intuitively to seek out the stone most able to help. It could be colour, texture, or feel, or what I myself know to be the indefinable something that tells you it is right. She explained that crystals are minerals but some minerals did not have an external crystal form. All minerals had healing properties, each having its own individual and specific energy. Minerals could help us to direct and focus our energy.

Stones had more power in their natural state and keeping some loose near to you in the corner of a pillow in bed or held in the hand during relaxation or meditation, Lesley said, was beneficial to healing. Often they were put into a handbag or used as an ornament or in jewellery but Lesley said that I was correct in thinking that the more proximate to the person in their natural form the better the healing qualities.

I said that I had had for many years two rings set in silver—one a rose quartz and one malachite – green being my favourite colour – and that I always felt an uplift when wearing them. Lesley agreed that it could have been their healing qualities or just that the colours appealed to me. Either way I didn't mind just as long as I benefited. I explained that I had never needed a factual or scientific answer to anything . If it felt right, and my instincts were invariably sound, then this satisfied me. I was just grateful to have found a new healing power.

On looking around the shop I found many stones new to me. A large septarian concretionary grey module of clay iron-stone cut in half, showing it intersected within by cracks filled with calcite, dominated one corner of the shop, whilst on another shelf were small boxes containing restful prayer beads, which could be used to aid concentration and as Lesley volunteered, for saying a mantra, something simple and often in sanskrit which could bring about peace.

I held a large surprisingly heavy piece of rock crystal of obelisk shape, which was so cold to the touch and so well resembled a block of ice that I appreciated that this would not only make an unusual ornament, but have a cooling effect on frayed nerves. Just holding it, I could feel a calm serenity enveloping me.

Lesley said that they had over seventy different stones from all over the world, some more difficult to obtain than others, and I was eager to see and feel ones that appealed to me. My birth stones were carnelian or moonstone and Lesley put a selection before me. The carnelian was a thick ruddy brown colour which Lesley explained had a passionate and fearless energy. Traditionally it was associated with circulation and blood flow, the stone of blood ties and motherhood. It had the energy of a mother's instinctive and fearless protection of her children, or a warrior's self-assured independence. It was useful for the relief of congestion and tension. I held the stone in its polished state and it was warm and comfortable in my hand. In its natural state it was rough but still had a warm quality that I liked. The moonstone was entirely new to me and I perceived an almost ephemeral quality about it as I turned the polished stones in my hand, that in one instant were transparent and in another held a brief glimpse of milky hue, so subtle that it was hardly there. This stone was cooler than the carnelian and I found it good to hold. In its natural state it was a light white grey, with a hint of pale brown that blended in harmony with the carnelian. It was associated with emotions and family ties and was connected with the moon, the sea, and with time – the ebb and flow of life. It had the energy of cool, gently flowing water. When emotional temperatures were running high, this stone had a cooling effect. It was like a safe harbour or a port in a storm. I was well satisfied that one of my birthstones was associated with water as I had an instant rapport with any lake, river, waterfall and of course the all encompassing sea. I did feel that both of these stones could be advantageous to me. Lesley explained that stones kept in a pocket would be passive but when held in the hand became active.

To obtain maximum advantage from mineral stones I knew that I had to give it my total concentration. To sit in a quiet room of even temperature, holding the stone lightly or placed within easy eye range or just beside me I found best. To sit and breathe evenly, letting everything drift away and becoming only conscious of the stone and its health-giving properties, I would sit with my eyes closed, aware of the stone in my hand as I breathed in its goodness. The stillness encompassed me and as peace descended the stone melted into my hand and became an integral part of me, as its cognisant mineral energies coursed through me. Such was the latent power of the stone. Sometimes I would place it near to me – look at it before closing my eyes so that I was aware of its shape, density and colour, and visualise the power flowing from it into me. If its clarity faded I looked at it for an instant before again closing my eyes. Doing this only for a short time I found helped renew energy and to regain a feeling of serenity and well being . Having been a willing exponent of all natural healing methods for a long period, I welcomed this new one into my life.

I looked further around the shop in search of a favourite stone and found it – the peridot – the nonpareil. To gaze into its endless green depths is like diving into the sea, down and down to be filled with a refreshing verdancy until it is all around you and in you, and you are part of the flickering sparkling depths, until you emerge, envigorated and full of clarity of spirit. The first peridot stone that I had ever seen was on holiday with my cousin Jan's family when we were children, and in the old stone cottage nestling against a mountain hollow in Meirionnydd, we would spend dark evenings showing each other our treasures. Jan had a ring in which was set a peridot as green as a piece of captured sea. I would place it on my finger and turn it in all directions and gaze at the differing inflections. It was so alive that I could sense and smell the sea in it. It is described as having the energy of being near a cool pool in the woods where the animals go to drink at dawn and at dusk. This is the stone of intuitive understanding, of the need to go beyond what is seen as good or bad. I know that this stone will always have importance for me.

Over the years I have collected pebbles from the beach at Criccieth. At first glance the beach is just a mass of grey stones, but on looking closer you can find unusual pebbles of all shapes and sizes and in varied colours – some with gentle complimenting shades and others with stark dramatic contrasts. I now have many. In my bedroom is one of a delicate green shade that brings peace when I look at it. Is it because it is my favourite colour, because it is from the place that I love so well, or does it have healing qualities? I don't know, but I feel good about it and the other stones, so maybe there is some hidden secret waiting to be found in them. Whatever it is they are sufficiently important for me not to be parted from them.

I was grateful for the time given to me willingly by Lesley and was reluctant to leave her shop of delights, but I promised to return again.

When I again visited "Wyvern" it was with pleasurable anticipation of time to be spent in a small place full of vibrant energy, and of course, I was eager to meet Chris. Just as Lesley had, she gave me a warm welcome, and I was soon ensconced in a chair surrounded by the display shelves bidding me look at their wares. I gave a quick look at the stones now familiar to me, as always the green ones holding my gaze momentarily, before I concentrated on Chris. Like Lesley she seemed calm and serene and full of quiet authority – all that I wanted to be, and I eagerly plied her with questions that she willingly answered.

She explained that as well as being a partner with Lesley she also held meetings for interested persons to learn more about healing with crystals. Natural crystals, minerals and gemstones harmonised with the emotions and could be used as stepping stones along the path to greater acceptance. She also gave private hourly consultations. Both crystals and counselling were used in these sessions to help resolve emotional conflicts arising from personal problems, (illness and many more), including a lack of creativity in life. The consultations were based on holistic therapy, centring on emotions as aspects of the personality.

Healing with stones took time for results, just like with any other therapy. I soon realised that just because it was such a novel idea for me did not mean that it did not achieve the desired results. She used the stones to balance the energy system. If the imbalance in the emotional state were corrected, this would in turn assist in correcting the physical imbalance. Homoeopathic medicines were often minerals and this would be the same in content as a specific stone. I just had to get used to a different way of the medicine being administered – instead of the usual pill taken orally it was the proximity of a stone to the body, the mineral content being exactly the same. Chris explained that in some countries it was natural for stones to be used in healing. We in the more sophisticated "enlightened" countries had for many years now waived aside these remedies, but many more people were now realising the healing powers of these methods, and were willing to return to our natural roots, and learn to be healed as our ancestors had been.

Like all medicines, healing with crystals had its own "first aid" for initial use before more specific use of stones might be prescribed.

> Rock crystal (also known as clear quartz) was used to help relieve stress and for stillness.

> Amethyst was used for pain and helped with nervous disorders as it helped regain serenity.

> Banded Agate was used for people inclined to worry. I did know that this was a talismanic stone which

when worn as an amulet would guard its wearer from all dangers.

Rose Quartz helped stabilise emotions.

Blue Lace Agate was used to help the healing energy activate in the body.

These remedies were beneficial to everyone.

Chris and Lesley explained to me how different areas in the country had different minerals due to varying rock structures. I mentioned my beach pebbles to them, and they said these would be a mixture of minerals, and I was gratified to learn aided healing. This made me also feel that the limestone where I lived could transfer its powers to me, and it would be so easy for me to obtain some.

I asked whether the more precious stones like diamonds, rubies and emeralds were as conducive to healing. Chris explained that they were also minerals and therefore could be used but were not normally. These stones were invariably cut and set and sold as jewellery. The cutting stresses the stone. Diamonds were the hardest and brittle and therefore more likely to crack when cut. Unlike other stones they were subject to the regulations of the diamond cartel which only allowed cut stones to be imported. Although I appreciated the brilliance of these precious gems they had never held much appeal to me with their showy hard glitter. I much preferred the less exotic mellow stones with which I now found myself surrounded. As I now already knew, stones in their most natural form held the greatest healing powers. Chris also explained that stones can crack when used for healing and this was more likely when they had already been cut. She also said that she used jewellery herself for healing, using the most appropriate stones at any particular time. I had noticed the attractive neckless that she was wearing of bright alternate colours; these being, turquoise, jet and mother of pearl. She said that as she had a number of stones together these were less likely to fracture than when just a single stone was used. I told her that it had been recommended that turquoise would help me by Marilyn, a colour therapist, and Chris said that the stone would also help if this was the colour diagnosed as being most needed by me.

I asked whether crystals deteriorated or lost potency with age, and Lesley informed me that the majority of stones, if cared for and kept clean, would retain their healing powers indefinitely. Some stones of a softer consistency could become damaged, like opals, and the turquoise absorbed grease over a period of time. Conversely, the quartz was a hard crystal and would never deteriorate.

With all this knowledge whirling around in my head I reacquainted myself with the treasures on display, which included my old friends the warm golden iron pyrites, deep reassuring malachite and palest rose quartz, so delicate that it was the faintest rosy blush that the slightest puff of wind would blow away.

New stones caught my attention. Sphalerite (also known as blende or zinc blende, had a somewhat bright but non-metallic lustre) on calcite was a white opaque stone with brown-beige inflections and was reminiscent of luscious lumps of crumbly vanilla fudge, it was so edible in appearance. I was interested to see that it came from Tankerville in Shropshire where a special family friend Peter had once owned the Tankerville Arms. He is an unusual, fascinating and well travelled person and I like to think of him living near to this mellow stone.

Barytes (also known as heavy spar) also from my favourite County Shropshire, was white, and made me think of marble as it was luminous and felt quite heavy, but friendly. This was placed near to the contrasting red jasper which was an amorphous variety of quartz stained predominantly red brown with green and yellow. The stone that I held in my hand was a dull warm colour, light to hold and reassuring.

The minty mottled effect of green aventurine which is a translucent quartz, spangled throughout with scales of mica or other mineral, I particularly liked, and the blue lace agate egg from Kenya, which was a variegated chalcedony polished and glossy in pale blue grey with cloud-like formations interwoven in marshmallow. Its webb inspired tracings caused a waft of sad music to enter my mind for a fleeting moment.

Already I was subconsciously thinking of the effects the different stones had on me and I accepted that they could and would heal. I was happy to have met Lesley and Chris and grateful for all that they had told me. I now had to learn how to put it all into use, and I realised how much fun I should have experimenting with these stones and making them work for me.

It suddenly dawned on me that there was a wealth of information here on my own doorstep in the geological section of our excellent museum. This we had visited many times over the years, but never with our recently acquired knowledge, and it was with impatience that I waited for the first afternoon that Brian, Jamie and myself were free to furnish our minds with deeper understanding. We were the only visitors to the relevant department, which was as well, due to my exclamations at seeing so many new stones as well as recognising the ones with which I was well acquainted. Initially I tried to look at everything in my wish to absorb all that I could of these geological phenomena – some of which were millions of years old – until the rule of order and method took over as being the sure way of not missing anything.

A whole afternoon passed swiftly due to my unbounded interest in these unusual minerals, and I examined the items familiar to me first. There was iron pyrites, which is a naturally occurring ore, containing iron sulphide crystals of which I had a piece at home. This specimen was nothing like it, not so golden and bright, but with small pieces of it which were embedded in thin strands on a dull flattened piece of black shale, which was a fissile rock formed by the consolidation of clay mud or silt having a finely stratified or laminated structure and composed of minerals essentially unaltered since deposited.

There was amethyst impregnated deep in iron ore with its colour ranging in varying shades of clear purple to bluish violet. A crystallised quartz was a lustrous finding partially hidden in its dark protective casing, and I was interested to see that it had come from Somerset. At home I placed a piece of natural amethyst close by a handful of fallen copper beach leaves that I had collected. The stone gleamed a deeper hue and the leaves took on a purple silver tone as the ensemble glistened in a shaft of sunlight.

Gleaming copper bright bronze shines as a new penny with its smooth bubbling bonded with the palest sage colour that is instantly recognisable.

In the show cases were many pieces new to me and I was riv-
ited by a small case that was filled with kaleidoscopic bril-
lance. For the first time I gazed upon fluorescent minerals.
These glowed when exposed to ultraviolet light which like X-
rays is invisible to us, as it has a short wave-length but fluorescent minerals can absorb it and give off visible light in
exchange. Fluorspar was the first mineral made to glow under
ultra-violet light – hence the word fluorescent. It was usually
blue or yellow but in ultraviolet light could glow blue, yellow
or green. Often the same colour fluorspar can glow different
colours as can other minerals. White calcite could glow red,
pink, green, yellow or blue. White scapolite could glow bright
yellow or orange. Willemite glowed a radiant green, whilst
sodalite was a glorious peach with interspersed blotchings of
pale purple.

I turned from this luminiferous case to other new stones
beckoning me. The snowflake obsidian with such an appropriate name was as shiny as high grade coal with abstract white
skitters and was actually volcanic glass, so unusual that it
hardly seemed credible that it was a natural phenomenon.

Gypsum or satin spar was the purest white with the satin
glazing of mother of pearl in parts, so clean and virginal that
it seemed impossible that this could have emanated in the
darkest earth.

Similar in name but a million miles apart in appearance
and texture was the gypsum desert rose which came from
Tunisia. It resembled rich toffee, which made the mouth
water and was structured in waxy petal shapes.

Another new stone that captured my interest, initially, as it
came from a favourite holiday haunt of ours – Aberdyfi – was
the chalcopyrite, a yellow copper-iron sulphide which was a
solid warm golden glow and a friendly stone.

Totally dramatic was the generous sized lemon sponge
looking sulphur, which was a non-metallic element occurring
naturally, encrusted with a profusion of glowing slivers of
celestite.

The opulent warmth of the brown-orange of the citrine
(burnt amethyst) could practically be felt when near, and with
its crystallisation was like an invitation to autumn.This complemented the orpiment nearby, a crystalline mineral with its
similar colouring.

As always, stones of any shade of green attracted me. There were a number of new ones with subtle variations on what I considered my colour. The dioptase (copper emerald), a hydrous copper silicate, was an opaque glow of darkest hue.

The wavellite was a mixture of damp mossy green with honey beige and palest grey, and of thick density, that to look upon it was to dive fathoms down into the deepest ocean.

The hemimorphite from Mexico was the palest aqua-marine, striking by its smoothness, spread across a light textured rock like icing on a cake.

The inscrutable black smoky quartz was a dramatic collection of sinister dark glossy dagger shapes, which contrasted evilly with the delicate silver white spines of the needle quartz.

I learned that minerals were the raw materials from which rocks were made. There were over two thousand different types and they were all categorised according to their properties. These included colour, crystal form, lustre or shine, hardness, specific gravity and the way the mineral cleaved or fractured.

Certain minerals were valuable because they had special properties. Gem stones had long been used for jewellery because they had rich colours and could be cut to display a shining lustre. The most popular gemstone, diamond, was the hardest substance known and was also used for cutting or grinding other materials.

Ore minerals were perhaps the most important of all. From these we got such metals as iron, copper, lead and zinc. The most precious metals are the rarest and most enduring ones; gold, silver and platinum. All were used in jewellery, but had other applications as well as in electronics and the manufacture of coins.

I came home feeling on the highest cloud. I had found the world of geology. Every day I was learning of so many spheres of life hitherto untapped by me that I eagerly turned to.

Jamie casually announced that I had no need to search for crystals as he could make me a variety of crystals of varying shapes, sizes and colours. I looked at him in disbelief as he said nothing, but went upstairs to where he kept his library. I could hear him rummaging about and eventually he staggered downstairs weighted down with three enormous tomes. With a flourish he placed them before me, opened at the appropriate chapter and I read of synthetic crystals. These were grown by a variety of processes from the appropriate chemical ingredients, and had the same chemical composition, internal crystal structure and physical properties as their natural counterparts – where they existed. Many thousands of solids were crystalline, but the expression synthetic crystals was usually understood to refer to the few hundred crystals, all difficult to make, which were of considerable value either to industry or as gemstones, or, frequently both. If they had natural equivalents, these would mostly have been formed millions of years ago from hot molten liquids, cooling under pressure when the earth was forming. All the important and valuable gemstones had been synthesised, including diamonds, rubies, saphires and emeralds, but they had only a fraction of the commercial value of their natural counterparts. All except emerald had industrial uses. Diamonds were the last of the crystals to be made artificially and these did not have the bright transparency of natural diamonds but a duller more amber colour. I read with interest about growing crystals, which Jamie had so nonchalantly promised to do for me. Crystallisation occurs from a solution of molten salt or vapour. The crystal grows by the addition of a new material until an equilibrium is reached when the rate of deposition of material equals the rate at which the crystal was dissolved into the surrounding medium. Crystallisation normally took place when a concentrated solution is cooled. In some cases it was necessary to 'seed' the solution with a minute particle of the solid. This particle formed the nucleus around which crystals grew. Jamie proceeded to do this for me with copper sulphate and I am now the proud possessor of a petri dish of home made crystals of the clearest cyan. The light diffuses as I turn the dish about causing the crystals to give out silver bright lights. Whatever crystals I may be fortunate enough to possess in the future, none will be as precious as these made specially for me. I asked Lesley whether these crystals that Jamie had made for me would be as beneficial for healing purposes as the natural counterparts, as, quite correctly, Jamie had pointed out to me that they contained the same elements. She said that she thought that there would probably be some difference, but she had never sought out any and felt that she would prefer to work with natural stones. She was interested in what I had said and agreed to experiment with such stones should the occasion arise. She also confirmed to me that the elements found in crystals were the same as those in plants and would therefore contain the same amount of goodness. Obviously food gives immediate benefit when eaten and healing by crystals would take longer but this whole concept was fascinating to me.

From the time of my birth I had been fortunate enough to have an Aunt Nellie who thought young ladies should wear what she called "good jewellery". Each Christmas my cousins Jan, Jo and I had been given suitable gifts, only differing in our initials engraved on appropriate pieces, and we accepted it as normal to have an impressive number of such items. It was only in later years that we realised how fortunate we were, and that our knowledge of jewellery had commenced in such a personal way. Jan particularly enjoyed adding to her collection by her own choice, often purchased when on holiday, when I would join in its appreciation with her. We had an unusual childhood in many respects, but it gave us insights to many things unknown to most children.

I also read that many rocks in the earth's crust were carbonates. Three were chalk, limestone and marble. Chalk was first formed in the sea. The shells of sea-animals consisted of calcium carbonate. When the animals died the shells sank to the bottom of the sea. After thousands of years the shells formed a layer of chalk. If other rocks covered the chalk, great pressure changed it to limestone. Pressure and heat on limestone changed it to marble. The changes were physical, and all three rocks were calcium carbonate. Coral, pearl and many shells contained calcium carbonate. The carbonates of zinc, iron, lead and copper occurred naturally. Limestone was of particular interest to me as I was always surrounded by it. Living in a limestone area meant that I was always proximate to a natural mineral substance that I had never given a thought to as I had lived close to it all of my life. It was soft and crumbly and on exploring the long disused workings of mines, I always thought it a rather sad, lonely shade of grey, but mellow and friendly, and had always liked it. Touching it it is warm and its powder dusts my hands. I like it. It is part of my birthright and not to be discarded as it is a mineral and must have healing qualities. Just because it was not used therapeutically did not mean that I must refrain from doing so. It is not on sale in "Wyvern", nor have I ever seen it on sale anywhere. This does not bother me, in fact it makes it more special to appreciate it and besides, a dish of it beside the one Jamie has given me makes me feel good.

My awareness and interest in crystallography, geology and the healing property – plus obvious beauty – of stones all seemed to be linked and could loosely be called natural science. Had I really said when young that I disliked science? I know that I had. It was a case of ignorance causing me to make a stupid statement. Science is a fascinating subject and I had only made the tiniest scratch on its surface. I shall always be grateful to Lesley and Chris of "Wyvern"for opening my eyes and seeing life in a new way and welcoming me so warmly into their world.

Hypnosis

Often the best things in life come to us unexpectedly and meeting Jaki was one of those occasions. She swept into my life like a friendly whirlwind and shook me out of my complacency and encouraged me to think in a way that I never had before. She was so full of life that you could almost see the electricity emanating from her and her contentment with life was obvious. She was all that was magnanimous, and when she told me that all her life all that she had wanted to do was help people, I realised how fortunate I was to have met her.

She taught me many things. She said that I gave too much of myself to others and became emotionally and physically drained, and must learn to put on a protective shell to stop this happening. She suggested imagining putting myself into a sack and pulling it up around me, and then tying it at the top. This would help to contain my own energy, and also stop it being taken away by others, and, important for me, help me to cope better. Cleansing my home would also lift my spirits, not that she was suggesting that it was dirty – more to shake away the dull and dead thoughts, and make it lighter and brighter and a happier place to be in. This in turn would help restore my feeling of well-being. As others had already told me, she said that I must learn to love myself more before I could love others.

One day, when a number of members of Dudley Group were talking we mentioned fears, and Georgina, one of the helpers at the Group, volunteered a lifelong dread of visiting the dentist and how she had overcome this. As I also disliked dental visits I was interested in her solution. Georgina viewed the world through cool blue eyes and was a quietly spoken almost reticent person, but when she did speak what she had to say was invariably worth listening to. She explained how in 1989 she had taken a short course of six sessions of hypnosis to alleviate her fear, and that this had been so successful she never had any reluctance to visit the dentist at any time since. This statement I found quite incredible to believe, but she assured her listeners that it was true.

When Jaki said that she was a hypnotherapist and that she was sure that she could help me I was dubious, as I had always viewed this as more of a magic show than of therapeutic value. However, as Georgina was proof that this did work, when I looked into Jaki's open encouraging face I agreed to have a session with her.

The origins of hypnosis remain unclear, but it was used as a cure method by civilisations such as the ancient Egyptians, Persians, Greeks and Romans. In ancient communities it was even considered divine, because of the seemingly miraculous cures that could be effected while the patient was in such a state. The belief in the power of suggestion continued in the Middle Ages, spreading through Europe and Britain.

One of the first people who claimed to use hypnosis as a cure was an Austrian doctor, Franz Anton Mesmer (1734-1815) who was reputed to have worked at the court of Queen Marie Antoinette, famed in history books by the words attributed to her *"Let them eat cake"* when she was told that the starving people of France had no bread. Mesmer was something of a showman and reading about his techniques gives us a clue as to why hypnotism has the reputation it does today. He wore silk robes, and a wand and used heavily perfumed rooms. He was basically a sincere healer and believed that the cure was due to an invisible, magnetic substance, which had rebalancing effects through his fingers and wand. He was eventually pronounced a fraud by a specially appointed Medical Committee. The concept of "animal magnetism" as it became known, was continued by the only people who could take it along the path where it was then directed – conjurors and magicians. Mesmer retired in obscurity, yet his name remains today in the word mesmerism and inspired others to delve into hypnotism.

The word 'hypnosis' was coined by James Braid in 1843, a Scottish surgeon who revived the use of mesmerism for some of his operations. During Victorian times, hypnotism once more caught the attention of medical men, and it also gained ground after the first world war, when it was used to help alleviate the symptoms of wartime traumas. Since then there has been a gradual, cautious acceptance of it, but it has never acquired the credibility of other natural therapies.

I remembered the only time that I had come into contact with hypnosis before it was now mentioned by Jaki. When I was a small girl on an annual summer holiday in Llandudno with my parents and Aunt Ada, we had sat in the Happy Valley and gazed down onto the stage of the open air theatre at the base of the Great Orme where a fascinated audience watched a show which included a magicians act. Members of the audience were invited to assist and there were always many willing helpers. Some would sit on chairs, and after being put into a hypnotic trance would do as directed by the hypnotist. Some would "eat their dinner" and I remember one person being requested to "give some to his cat" which he proceeded to do by removing an imaginary morsel from his plate. Another appeared to be suspended above the ground on nothing but air. I recalled now these long forgotten memories and with some trepidation and caution wondered how Jaki would view this subject, which seemed more show business than medicinal.

Jaki duly arrived on the appointed day, as always her eager fresh face wreathed in smiles. She did not know how much I was in need of her help on that day, as on the evening prior to her visit I had had water gushing from a tap that I had been unable to turn off, and in desperation I had pleaded with my plumber Peter to help me. Recognising my need for his aid, he had postponed a family outing to dinner, and within a short time had solved my problem until he had time to fix the necessary new tap. I was appreciative of his immediate help, but the event had caused me to be in the slightly stressful state that would give Jaki something tangible to work on.

After an initial friendly chat Jaki suggested that we begin and said that she wanted me to position myself comfortably in a semi-upright chair, placing cushions in the small of my back and behind my neck. This was to give my body support as I became relaxed so that afterwards I would not suffer from any stiffness. My feet were to be placed flat on the floor and uncrossed. She was insistent that I did not lie down as she did not want me to fall asleep, but to be totally awake, as the hypnotic state is one of deep relaxation when one is completely conscious. It actually lies somewhere between sleeping and being awake, where all the subject's physiological reflexes are still present. A person is put into relaxation by an induction; this is something like the half-awake, half-asleep state you reach just before finally dropping off to sleep and when first waking up in the morning.

Jaki explained that the aim of hypnosis was to help alleviate stress, strain and physical ailments and to try to improve health on a one to one relationship between patient and therapist. Feelings, fears and phobias were brought into the open when in an altered state of consciousness. Approximately eighty per cent of people can be put into a light trance; a much smaller percentage will go into a deep trance. Jaki agreed with me that it was a great help if there was a rapport between the patient and therapist, and knowing the problems of the person requiring help, and the type of person, would assist in gaining the most benefit from the hypnotic state. Jaki knew that most of all I wanted to relax myself generally, as I knew that this was the way to help myself most of all.

Ascertaining that I was quite comfortable she asked me to focus on an object – any object of my choice and not to deviate my gaze from it, while I was to listen to her and do as she instructed. I chose a green plant in my rear garden, highlighted as it stood in the sunshine. She said that she would count upwards from one to ten and during that time my eyes would become heavy and I would close them, but only when I was ready. If my gaze wandered from my chosen object I was to bring it back to it whilst continuing to listen to Jaki's words. As it was early in the afternoon and the room was bright with sunlight, I was wide awake and, wanting to participate to the full, did not think that I would voluntarily close my eyes. Jaki asked me to relax – first from my toes and into my feet.

Relaxation always started from the feet as all goodness flowed from the earth and then travelled up and around the whole of the body. Jaki's words were interspersed with the number one and then two and I continued to fix my gaze on the plant, aware of the butterflies around it. The sun seemed to go less bright and I blinked my eyes. I became more aware of Jaki's quiet but authoritative voice as she continued the relaxation up through my legs and into my body – all the time continuing counting. By the time she had reached seven I closed my eyes that at her instruction had become heavy and I felt pleasantly drowsy. By the time she had reached number ten my eyes were firmly closed and my body totally relaxed and all my attention was on Jaki's voice. She told me that I was at all times in control, which I found reassuring.

I was not aware of my body at all – it just was not part of me – only my mind was completely alert as Jaki instructed me to look with my mind's eye and be aware of someone being massaged. Willingly I did as she directed, and at the same distance from me as the plant on which I had been focusing, I now saw a table with a masseur leaning over an inert figure. The figure was slim and dark haired and I realised that I was looking at myself. Jaki asked me to watch the figure being massaged and be aware of the sensations being experienced. My mind savoured the smooth movements over the back, easing the tension in the neck and shoulders and giving total relaxation. Mentally I pampered myself with the luxury of the massage, aware of the detachment of myself from reality but fully appreciating the soothing hands lightly caressing my body. Time stopped while I was in this limbo state that I had never been in before, totally aware of mental perfection in relaxation when I became conscious of Jaki's voice penetrating this picture of subliminal paradise. She said that she would count from one to five when I would become awake again. I listened to her voice with reluctance and as I opened my eyes and looked at her she was amused to see the cross look that I had given her. Where Jaki was concerned my eyes were the windows of my soul and in her astute way she could, without effort, read me as easily as a book. It had only seemed for a fleeting moment that I had been in a relaxed state but Jaki assured me that it had been for nearly half an hour.

With some shock I realised that there had been nothing

theatrical or unsavoury about hypnotherapy and that this was to me akin to relaxation and meditation – different but in harmony with them but entering into a deeper penetrating state of awareness. Jaki asked how I felt and I could truthfully say that I felt great. I was completely relaxed and the mental massage had made my body supple and totally free of stiffness and it had all ended much too soon.

Jaki told me that she had learned hypnotherapy some eight years ago and used it to gain access to another person's level of awareness, and in so doing help them in the way that they needed. The technique that Jaki used on me was suggestive hypnosis. With curative hypnotherapy the inductions were the same and the trust between therapist and patient were the same, but finding the cause to cure the symptoms that manifest themselves were slightly different, and this could be a lengthy process. She said that she wanted to perform miracles and in her so special way I knew that she could. She was absolutely fabulous.

Massage

If we are honest I think that all of us can benefit from some form of escapism. Something that takes us into a world that is as different as can be from the one that we live in, we find fascinating. I am no exception to this, and a favourite of mine has to be the larger than life world of James Bond. Everything that 007 comes into contact with is razor sharp with excitement, but nothing ruffles the suave good humour of this tongue-in-cheek character, and so his escapades are never frightening, but first class entertainment to the average housewife and mother like myself. To sit comfortably in the familiar warmth of my own sitting room near the fire on a cold winter evening with a tempting snack within arms reach and watch one of these films where the settings are the most exotic, the sun more brilliant and the action so stimulating, fills me with satisfaction. We watch the stars walk on a silver white beach, more beautiful than in other films with tanned limbs, dark and supple, and then we enter the luxurious hotel with tables loaded with Caribbean delicacies that James Bond never samples, but inevitably finds time for that most glorious relaxative affiliated to the aristocratic and the rich – the massage. Always appearing so sublimely sensual and deliciously decadent, I have always wistfully wanted to be the person on the table being helped to unwind in this so intimate way.

As probably the oldest therapy known to man, massage has been practised in the Middle and Far East for thousands of years. Physicians in ancient Greece were skilled in massaging stiff and painful joints and Hippocrates, known as "The Father of Medicine", wrote in the fifth century before Christ *'The way to health is to have a scented bath and an oiled massage each day'*.

Physically, massage is aimed at improving the blood, muscular and nervous systems, and also helping the body to assimilate food and get rid of waste products.

Mentally, on a psychological and emotional level, its calm and soothing effects have helped anxious people – allowing them to deal more constructively with everyday worries – and to regain self confidence.

Massage is also an extension of the basic human need to touch and be touched, and one of the most humane therapies in the world. It can be used to improve general well-being and reduce stress – and for me this was its most appealing aspect, being my personal bogey – and of course it brings the close and sympathetic contact with another human being.

I was delighted when Marilyn offered to give me a massage. She did however point out that any cancer patients or anyone undertaking medical treatment should consult their doctor before having a massage. As always she arrived with a heavy load. For a small person she was constantly struggling with mountainous equipment, but with Jamie's help we soon had all the items that she needed in my sitting room, now dominated by her table. She drew the curtains, not only for privacy, but for the peace that a darkened room can give and as she started to play a tape of haunting peaceful music and lit a candle,the room took on a new dimension of a spiritual nature that was present in all of the healers that I had had the pleasure of meeting.

Marilyn explained to me that over a period of time the result of imbalances in the body's energies can cause illness, although some can be hereditary. Our thoughts and feelings can also affect our health, causing stress, and I knew only too well how true her words were.

I undressed and lay on the table, quite relaxed, as I trusted

Marilyn to help me in another of her gifted ways, but alert and expectant of what was to come.

Initially she lightly put oil of lavender and geranium on my body, which made it easier for her to massage it, and was good for the skin. The lavender oil relaxed the muscles.

She went up and down my spine with circular movements. The pressure stimulates circulation and enables joints to move more freely. She then went over my shoulders and body generally before lightly massaging my legs and feet. By this time I was hardly concentrating on what she was doing, just giving myself totally to this blissful feeling of the whole body being supple and free of tension all over, and savouring every precious second of it. I felt almost a sense of timelessness as my relaxation increased.

At her request I obediently turned into different positions as she flexed my arms to release tension. She massaged my stomach which was so novel to me and so unusual that I could not refrain from laughing, but it was pleasurable in the strange sensations that emanated from her fingers and spread through the whole of my lower body.

Gently but firmly she massaged the top of my spine up into the commencement of my hair which was an area of tension for me and it was absolute ecstacy to feel her searching fingers massaging all the stiffness away. Turning my head to one side she gently pulled it, first on one side and then the other. This was done to eradicate stiffness. I lay supine, lethargically moving as asked by Marilyn and now luxuriously relaxed beneath her hands. I could feel the love waves that she exuded penetrating my flesh and filling me with pure goodness. She was a person full of sunshine and so eager to share herself with others who needed her help.

Finally her hands flowed over the length of my body but not touching it, and I could feel the current drawn to the flow of her hands. Marilyn explained that this was to straighten out the magnetic field.

I was disappointed when it was over, and wanted to start again from the beginning, but I felt indescribably at peace and invaded with a warmth that filled my bones, and I knew that I had been right in my thinking over so many years that I would find massage an inspiration and that I would want to participate in it as often as I could. For me it was the most enjoyable of all the natural therapies that I had been fortunate enough to experience. It had also fleetingly given me a glimpse of the world of the pampered Bond girls.

Marilyn said that basically I was relaxed, apart from my heart and stomach areas, which were heavy and needed a course of therapy. She said that I gave the appearance of being tense, but as I explained to her, this was only because I was so eager to be alert and to assimilate all that I could from her and so apply her knowledge to myself. .

Marilyn then asked me to sit upright on a stool so that she could balance my chakras. I sat in the dusk-filled quiet of the room, aware of my regular shallow breathing, as she moved her hands around my body, close, so that I was aware of her, but without touching me. She confirmed that basically I was physically relaxed, but as had been disclosed during my massage, my heart and stomach areas were heavy and needed to be healed. She suggested that I have my chakras rebalanced monthly to see how I was progressing.

I had previously heard of the chakras from a variety of people and they are explained in detail in the excellent small volume on colour healing by Mary Anderson, which gave me added insight to what I already knew.

The chakras are continually moving wheel-like vortices situated in the etheric body – the aura – a pattern on which the physical is built. The etheric body, the vital counterpart of the physical, is important as it draws in the life energy from the atmosphere and distributes it through the system. Disease begins in the etheric body before entering the physical and can therefore assist in an early diagnosis of impending disease. It is the first of the seven auras and ranges from the physical to the spiritual. Everyone has an aura and this consists of energy bands of colours of the spectrum. The ditty "Richard of York Gave Battle in Vain" is an easy way to remember the sequence of the rainbow colours of red, orange, yellow, green, blue, indigo and violet. These seven auras link up with the chakra centres situate down the body at definite intervals which again are governed by the colour spectrum.

The first centre is red; the lowest centre in the base of the spine and a physical element.

The second centre is orange; in the small of the back to the left-hand side of the spine (splenic area) and is a vitality element

The third centre is yellow; in the middle of the back over the kidneys (solar plexus area) and is a psychological element.

The fourth centre is green; between the shoulder blades in line with the heart and is a harmonising element.

The fifth centre is blue; at the base of the skull (throat centre) and is a specific healing element.

The sixth centre is indigo; in the forehead, the pineal gland (brow centre) and is an element of inspiration and intuition.

The seventh centre is violet; in the crown of the head (pituitary gland) and is a spiritual element.

As I had learned from Marilyn there was nothing new in colour healing, only our re-acceptance of its power. The Ancient Wisdom teachings identify seven major chakras along the spine and in the head. These wheels of rotating subtle matter represented energy centres. The organs of the body have affinity with each of these.

The red chakra controls the creative and reproductive system.

The orange chakra influences the process of digestion and assimilation.

The yellow chakra relates to imbalance in the adrenal glands, pancreas and liver.

The green chakra is the focus for diseases of the heart, the blood and circulatory system. Marilyn also informed me that green is the colour used for cancer control, but that like all medication it should be used in moderation as too much could destroy good cells.

The blue chakra is needed to treat diseases connected with the throat and thyroid glands and is located at the back of the neck.

The indigo chakra is found between the eyebrows. Diseases of the brain, eyes, nose, ears and nervous system are treated by focusing on this chakra.

The violet chakra is at the crown of the head and is needed to help those who are nervous and highly strung by nature. It is soothing and tranquillising and can help restore peace and calm.

I had gained benefit in the past from colour breathing, subconsciously using obvious colours like green for peace and blue for coolness. My body had shown me what to do long before I had been aware of colour healing. Red and orange gave warmth over the whole body and of course yellow, the colour of the sun, gave the all-fulfilling happiness ray. It is so easy to sit quietly, outside if possible, and I have found it advantageous, particularly after rainfall when all is fresh and clean and pleading to be used to aid good health. To sit in the green of my garden surrounded by many mature trees is to envelope myself in its richness in all weathers, just as to sit outside on a day full of sunshine has to cheer the heart. Sit and relax and expel all the air from the lungs and then gently and evenly fill your lungs with the colour that you require. Feel it lightly touching your face and your fingers, before being breathed into you and giving your body all of its goodness as it saturates your whole being. Do not force the breaths. Just do what feels comfortable and after five minutes you will notice the difference. Like everything else it requires practice but it is such a glowing way to help your body regain the balance that it needs with a therapy full of pleasure.

Finally, visualise happiness and good health and serenity and all of those different colours working in their own individual way and you will have learned how to participate in colour healing.

As I have repeated so many times always at the basis of any healing that I have devised for myself is correct diet and I was fascinated to learn that as well as the appropriate colour being used for a specific physical imbalance – food of the appropriate colour was also recommended.

Diet to help when the colour red was needed should include some of my favourite foods; cresses, black cherries, radishes and beet.

Diet to help when the colour orange was needed should include most orange skinned vegetables and fruits, apricots, peaches and carrots.

Diet to help when the colour yellow was needed basically consisted of yellow skinned vegetables and fruit and at the top of my list was the enzyme filled pineapple.

Diet to help when the colour green was needed included all the green fruits and vegetables that did not give an alkaline or acid reaction but were neutral, and the list of these was endless, as for years I had eaten many items of my favourite colour without realising this twofold benefit that I was obtaining.

Diet to help when the colour blue was needed included grapes and blackberries which were always part of my breakfast menu.

Diet to help when the colour indigo was needed was the same as for the colour blue.

Diet to help when the colour violet was needed should include purple grapes, blackberries, purple broccoli and beetroot. These last three colours are closely linked and an interchangeable diet can be used.

Hydrotherapy

Water in all its guises has fascinated me for as long as I can remember – from the crystal cascades of waterfalls in wild Wales to the stillness of a hidden reservoir high up in the mountains – from the lightest drizzle of rain to the relentless pounding of a stormy sea. Perhaps my affinity with all water was due to the fact that seventy to eighty per cent of the human body consists of water, as does the earth's surface or maybe I had always subconsciously been aware of the healing qualities of water from the invigoration I always felt after a walk in the rain.

When two of my friends at Dudley Group, Mary and Ethel, extolled the virtues of their weekly visits to the hydrotherapy pool at our local hospital, I was interested. They mentioned the warmth of the water, how peaceful and relaxing it was and how much they thought it would help me to unwind. When I told them that swimming had always been a favourite sport of mine, they were incredulous at my hesitancy. What they did not know was that it had been over twenty years since I had been in a pool of any kind. That last occasion had been a happy birthday celebration that Brian and myself had shared prior to a lavish meal at a hidden hotel in the heart of Shropshire and lazy hours spent in the sunshine of a hot day, interspersed with dips in the open air swimming pool. It had been one of those magical days when the only sound, apart from midsummer hum, had been our bodies cutting through the water and feeling the heat of the sun drying us as we lay beside the pool afterwards. Years had gone by and swimming had taken a backward step, and now since the diagnosis of my heart condition I was cautious of taking any risk. One day Ethel suggested that I contact Diane, the hydrotherapist and have a talk to her. This seemed excellent advice which I took and found her a most understanding person. She listened attentively as I explained all that I could, and that my general practitioner had recommended that I participate in all that I wanted to in life that I felt I could, and be guided by my own feelings as to what I could safely undertake. She said that she would be happy for me to join the weekly group if my doctor was agreeable and I arranged to visit the pool.

My initial visit was on an Indian summer day in September when the first hint of autumn chill in the early morning air and dampness of the lawns swiftly dispersed to give a hazy warm day with vivid blue sky. Ironically, neither Ethel nor Mary were able to come with me, and when Jamie volunteered to accompany and look after me I was grateful. Of all the people he was the one who instinctively knew how and when to help me and as he was a strong swimmer I felt fortunate to have such a capable and caring son. Never for a moment do I ever take for granted the special years when I am the centre of his world, for I realise that it will not be long before he is eager to carve his own life in an adult world, and this is as it should be. He carried our bathing suits and towels into the hospital that was filled with the saddest and most joyous memories for me – happy times when my career years had been spent within these mellow walls, and sad times when I had visited my mother after her unsuccessful operations. It felt strange to walk along those familiar corridors again, and it was a personal tragedy to me that this hospital was now under the threat of closure. We were directed into a building new to me and asked to sit until we were called to the pool. As we waited my nervousness increased; it was an emotional time for me. Swimming was the one joy I so wanted to participate in again and the one regret at not having done so for so long. As I sat with the little group now waiting, I turned to Jamie and was about to say that "perhaps we could just go home" when we were all called in and with pounding heart I followed the others. I had half imagined a room reminiscent of a steamy sauna and I was surprised to feel the coolness of the air as Diane, recognising me as the stranger in the group, came to meet me.

In spite of her youth I soon appreciated that she was a responsible person, and I listened carefully to all that she had to tell me. As it was my first visit she did not want me to stay in the pool for the hour allocated to us, but a short time only, and if in any way I felt unwell I was to let her know. She told me that the pool had been in use for approximately two years and was four meters by seven meters in size and that the water temperature was around thirty eight degrees Centigrade. She explained that for about ten minutes we would normally have gentle exercises and then for the remainder of our time we could stand, swim or float, using the aids placed around the edge of the pool to facilitate this, or just do as we pleased – enjoying the feel of the warm water soothing and healing our bodies. I had already learned previously from Diane that when in the water the effect of the buoyancy means that there was little weight going through the joints. The body weighed approximately ten per cent of the weight on dry land so movement was much easier. The warmth of the water relaxed the muscles and increased the circulation, so when exercising, the muscles could work better. The resistance given by the water also meant that it was possible to work hard without the effort of dry land exercises.

Like most of the therapies with which I was now becoming familiar, the idea of the external application of water to the body to stimulate a natural cure had also been in use since ancient times. A number of the ancient Greek temples were built at the sites of hot springs used for water healing in honour of Asklepios, the God of Medicine. Everyone knows of the hotsprings which have bubbled out of the ground for centuries at forty degrees centigrade which were used by the Romans at Bath, but these are unfortunately now decayed and not in use. The beneficial powers of water have a long tradition in Eastern Europe and Germany in particular, and in the

homoeopathic way are directed not at the obvious physical
disabilities and symptoms, but by treating the whole person.
The popularity and recognising of the idea that water is the
essence of life is growing, and in this country hydrotherapy
treatments can be obtained in many places, including the
famous baths of the spa towns of Droitwich and Leamington.

From earliest years I had been aware of the benefits of sea
water above all other, and the rubbery clinging seaweed I had
welcomed in the submerged rock pools that I had explored,
and I had felt its thick texture with my small enquiring fingers. I would float, trailing long pieces of brown weed, and as
I turned I made poetry in my movements in the water as it
curled around my body. The buoyancy of sea water always
exhilarated me, but I took care not to take an unwelcome
mouthful when an unsuspected wave covered my face. It was
only years later that I realised that in my childish fun with sea
and seaweed I was making my own version of thalassotherapy,
which recognised the powers of healing in seaweed and seawa-
ter.

Diane, satisfied that I could be relied upon to be the best
judge of any adverse reactions, invited me to enter the pool. I
walked down the steps with an attentive Jamie close behind
and stopped for an instant on a step when the water, surprisingly warm, lapped around my toes. I continued until my legs
and lower half of my body were submerged. I felt the pull of
the water as I walked slowly down, savouring the precious
moment of actually being in a pool again. I stood against the
side and holding the bar sank until only my head was above
water. I was aware of the water, soft and supportive with its
buoyancy, causing me to move gently like a boat at anchor in
a calm sea. Diane, keeping a close watch on me, asked how I
was and I truthfully said that I felt fine and she suggested that
I relax and just enjoy my first visit to the pool. I turned to
face the centre of the pool – Jamie close beside me – and he
asked whether I was going to swim to the other side? He could
not possibly know how nervous I was of doing this, but after so
many years of deprivation I knew that I could not possibly leave
without trying. He went across first and when he said that he
would save me should I be in danger of drowning, I relaxed, and
automatically took the first stroke. As I lifted my feet I could feel
the sympathy of the water, warm and comforting, and then as I

arched my back, the protest from muscles not used for many years. I was exultant. After so many years I had actually swum a few strokes, one of my aims during the years of illness, and now I had done it. The triumph was sweet. I stood at the side of the pool breathing quickly, aware of the gentle motion of the water against my skin, applauding my efforts and now apprehension was gone. I turned and held the bar so that none would be aware of the emotion which must be clearly etched on my face. As I became calm I allowed myself the luxury of blotting out all else but the satisfaction of being in this liquid life force, pushing against me like bands of oil until I was soothed. Without fear I loosed my hold on the side and lay back, feeling the water hold me secure as I raised my feet to float on my back – always my favourite position in water. I lay supine, almost lethargic, but fully aware of the wavelets gently massaging away all tension. I slowly moved my feet to bring me more horizontal and dipping my head further back until I was almost submerged, luxuriated in the water warmly caressing my cheeks. My body moved in perfect synchronisation as I floated free as a sea anemone, feeling the life-giving envigorating energy entering the whole of me from this perfect wetness. With all confidence restored I stood at the other side of the pool and jubilantly looked up into Diane's face and as I stood to speak to her I felt the water flow heavily from me and I sank to the more comfortable position just below the water. As I rested she explained that she did gentle arm and leg exercises that I felt were well within my capacity, but I accepted that she was wise in suggesting that I take it gently for this first visit. I contented myself with using the collar to float in the water, weightless now mentally and physically as I watched Jamie reminiscent of a leviathan as his strong strokes quickly took him across the small pool. I smile, thinking of his early attempts at swimming when he attended a beginners class with my friend Kath's daughter Rebecca. Jamie would gasp and flounder until not even his dark head was visible as he sank to the bottom. At that time he always seemed submerged. Conversely, blonde, dainty Rebecca hated to have her face wet and held it high in the water as she steered a course well away from everyone, like a glided graceful swan. How different they were, but how proud we mums were when they gained their first five metre badges. Jamie was now all confidence in the water and an expert swimmer so his encouraging comments to me now were sweet to my ears.

Gently swaying in rhythm with the water's movements, I was well content with my achievement, and as I closed my eyes and shut out the calm surroundings I was transported back in time to another swimming pool that was filled with children's shouts and laughter.from my early years I had been taken on regular visits to our local swimming baths with attentive and over-anxious mothers, with a group of school friends who also lived close by. The group always included my friend Linda, her brother Alfred and another boy Martyn. We had lots of fun together, but Martyn was always the best swimmer. I would watch enviously as he went up and down the baths with powerful strokes that I longed to emulate, but would tell him that he had an unfair advantage as he was the only one of us to have a pair of flippers. Sometimes this would have the desired result of me being allowed to borrow them, and I eagerly swam off – a few quick flicks of my feet taking me away from the group and giving me extra time to twist and turn in my childish make – believe world, when I became Lotte, the wife of Hans Hass, whose underwater romance had made such an impression on me. I would float in a sea of magic movement with hair streaming in the water as sharks swam around me, waiting to be rescued by my knight. I was brought back to reality by an undignified ducking from Martyn, and as I spluttered to the surface was forced to relinquish the precious flippers. After our swim we would hungrily devour the tomato ketchup sandwiches that we all relished, provided by our mothers, and then race to the shop upstairs for chocolate marshmallows. With our hair hanging damply around our shoulders we would fill our mouths quickly as we were called to "hurry" as it was time for the bus home. Our journey home was lively with the boys always denying knowledge of the pulls we girls suffered to our long plaits.

Always happy in close proximity to water of all kinds, I spent many happy Sunday mornings at Martyn's home where I was always made welcome by his parents, Carol and George. They were the only people that I then knew who had a garden pond. This fascinated me, and Martyn would point out the different species of fish that he had, and I soon became familiar with most of them – the oddly named sticklebacks, smooth newts and a variety of goldfish. I hid my fear of the frogs as no ten year old girl encourages being called a cissy. One warm summer day he allowed me to help clean out the pond, and I watched as he carefully transferred the fish into containers. In my anxiety to help I accidently lost some of the fish down the drain. He was cross with me and I was contrite – even then I would never deliberately harm anything living. However much I coaxed he was wise enough never to take me out in his canoe, but we did enjoy lots of good times together – mostly connected with water. I particularly enjoyed the times when I could persuade George, an accomplished musician, to play tunes on his accordion as I munched homemade cake, or the bonfire parties when we burned our mouths on hot jacket potatoes oozing butter onto our dirty fingers. Sometimes I was allowed to play with the electric train layout, which I much admired, and if a train did derail I could always blame their tabby cat Timmy, my feline ally. Throughout my childhood Martyn always looked after me, and on rare occasions when I needed any support I could always count on him to be there. As we grew older years went by and we never saw each other, so it was with gratitude on my part when he found the time from a busy life to help Jamie take his first faltering steps in becoming knowledgeable on his computer. Jamie always remembers this and the games and graphics discs that he gave to him, now many years ago, and he appreciated Martyn's kindness to him in a way that I certainly never did when I was young. I was jerked back to reality by Jamie anxiously holding my arm and asking, was I alright? Memories faded with the speed of a shutter closing as I looked up into his face and assured him that everything was just fine.

Instinctively I knew that it was time to bring my visit to a close and felt the water clinging to me, reluctant for me to depart, as I slowly climbed out of the baths. Diane suggested that I have a hot drink and lie down for half an hour as I would feel tired. I was surprised at this suggestion but as I looked around I saw the beds ready for use should they be needed, but I said I felt great, but would take her advice and have a lazy evening. We both dried and changed and Jamie rubbed my thick hair dry. Although he can be irritatingly forgetful he has always been protective of me and I am proud of this son who now towers over me.

I drove us home in a state of exhilaration and Jamie conceded that I had done well. This had been a momentous day. That evening I waited for any adverse reactions, but there were none. I consolidated the good that the visit to the hydrotherapy pool had given me by a warm bath followed by the usual warm spray from the hand held shower head, and then had an early night. My body felt warm and supple, with joints loose and free and mentally I felt good. I had overcome a tremendous hurdle in swimming these few strokes and I knew that not only was this visit I hoped the first of many, but also the precursor to me becoming again a regular swimmer at our local public baths.

Diane said she would be pleased to see me again and I knew how fortunate I was to have met another natural healer who would help me. Maybe it was because of my natural affinity with water or the tremendous boost to my confidence that this exciting day had given me, but I knew without a doubt that hydrotherapy was the favourite of all the natural therapies that I was now participating in and enjoying.

Metamorphosis

Many years ago I was told that the most precious thing that I had was my life and from that moment I did all that I could to ensure that I lived it to the full. Initially this was achieved by regaining and maintaining physical good health and then – more difficult – working on my mind until it was tuned to the highest degree of perception. Life is so all-encompassing that I strive to give it the ultimate satisfaction of total freedom, whilst at the same time being completely conscious of all that I am. I accept that life exists in some form even before conception and at the moment of conception all that was myself came into being. This has to be the most formative time of any life and when I met Margaret I knew that I had found someone who could help me clear any blockages which may have been set up in my pre-natal period.

Margaret is a charming lady of my own age with thick grey hair that I wish mine to emulate one day. At our first meeting I was aware of a certain detachment about her that was alien to all the therapists that I had previously come into contact with, but in no way did this make her unfriendly. She was different, and I wanted to know why. She was a reflexologist but this was not the reason for our meeting. She was also an exponent of the metamorphic technique about which I knew nothing. The dictionary definition of metamorphosis is change of shape, character, transformation and I was intrigued to know in what way she wished to change me.

She soon assured me that she had no wish to change me at all, but to act as a catalyst only, and would therefore remain totally centred and detached during metamorphic sessions in order to allow the recipients complete freedom to change in whatever way was right for them. I realised now why I had found her "different" – she was, and in a new and fascinating way for me. She wanted to help me without in any way imposing her will on me. The 'life force' or energy within me would take over and bring about the transformation which would enable me to fulfil my potential. The innate intelligence within me would know exactly what was needed to bring about this growth, evolution and movement out of my existing life.

When she told me that work was commenced on the feet, I enquired whether it was like reflexology with which I was familiar, and found most beneficial to health as well as enjoyable. She laughed and said it was nothing like reflexology and was in fact a step beyond it. This I found intriguing, but was to admit her words were true. The healing qualities of metamorphosis were almost intangible, but were waiting for anyone ready to progress to seek out and utilise for their own personal gain, health and happiness.

Margaret informed me that Robert St. John, an Englishman who was first a naturopath and a reflexologist, was the discoverer of the revolutionary approach to healing called metamorphosis. In the 1970's Gaston Saint-Pierre, a French Canadian born in 1940, trained with Robert St. John, and it was from him that Margaret had learned the metamorphic technique. He had told Margaret that everyone had an innate knowledge that knows what we need to achieve our potential and the metamorphic technique could remove blockages to our life force.

I realised that this was the most personal of the therapies that I was now to be initiated into, in that I would be the only person directing my own life energy. Margaret would assist almost as a liaisor or intermediary, but always detached, never in any way imposing her will, never directing or suggesting a way for me to go – only helping me to recognise how to heal myself in my own unique and perfect way.

The life force is split into three primary ways in which life manifests itself in man as energy, mind and emotion. These correspond to the physical structure of the body – hard and soft tissue and fluids. The hard tissue is the skeleton, the structure of our being and what we start life with. The soft tissue is the flesh, skin, nerves, muscles and organs and these represent the mental aspect and give us movement. The fluids are to me our secret life, the blood, water and lymph, which flow throughout our beings which change according to our emotions. The body is also split into three with the head (thinking) the hands (doing) and the feet (moving). The feet are the power of life and all important. The hands bring out the ability to do things. The head is for thinking and where initiative finds its source.

In the metamorphic way of life the spine is all important and the therapy is centred on the spinal reflexes that are found on the feet, hands and head. Margaret explained that all problems of a physical nature appeared along the foot spinal reflex. On an abstract level the spine reflex relates from the time before conception and also from conception to birth. At this time of development of the embryo and foetus, our present physical, mental, emotional and behavioural characteristics were established.

The right side of the body (left side of the brain) represented the masculine or giving, outward, logical side of our nature which we use daily. The left side of the body (right side of the brain) represented the feminine, receptive, intuitive, creative energy within us.

Margaret suggested that we commence my first self-healing with her, and I willingly extended my bare foot to rest lightly on a towel in her lap as she sat to the side of me for detachment. She always started with the right foot as this represented the present. This was explored with a firm touch, then the fingers were gently moved along the spinal and pelvic reflexes with light circling, vibrating or 'rain dropping' type movements. I was aware instantly of the calm warmth of Margaret's hands as they encircled my foot before lightly moving, soft as the sweetest caress until my whole foot and then body was responsive to her touch. Her voice drifted away but I was aware of her even tones as she continued to talk to me, but I could feel the power in my foot taking precedence over all else. My whole body felt warm and inviting and the top of my scalp tingled as if the lightest of needles were dancing as fairies in the morning dew of an enchanted field. Margaret continued for twenty minutes and then repeated the exercise on my left foot. On finishing either foot she stroked the foot downwards to ground me and finished the treatment at the heel. She then stroked in the aura.

The same treatment was then carried out on both hands, which was totally relaxing, as even though I suffered no stiffness of joints as my hands were poised for work for many hours a day – a great proportion on a typewriter – they were in a constant state of alertness and the treatment made them able to energise and bring out the latent life force in them.

The final treatment was on the head and this was bliss to me. My personal treat is the total relaxation found in having my hair brushed in all directions with a bristle brush, or massaged with gentle but firm fingers. Margaret's touch was a new experience, but one that raised me to a new plane of awareness. It was light and I was more conscious of her presence than her touch, and it was important not to drag at my hair or rearrange any hair style. Nothing must be done to try in the most innocent way to alter a persons personality or preference of choice. At the end of the treatment of the head the energy field was smoothed in a downward movement. This was refreshing for the patient and also regained calm.

Margaret said that on some people changes were almost immediately noticeable, but on others they were subtle. I assured her that I had gained from all the natural therapies in which I had been fortunate enough to participate, and the metamorphic technique was no exception. I was now completely relaxed after a mentally taxing morning that I had not envisaged or wanted, but nevertheless had happened, so she had completely annihilated any tension built, up and what was more important, she had acted as a catalyst and made me aware of how I could help my body help myself. I would happily go beyond all my present limits of awareness until unknown planes of ecstasy were reached.

I am glad that I did not learn of the existence of metamorphosis earlier in my life for I would not have been ready to understand it and therefore unable to accept it. It is not a therapy in the normal sense of the word, but more a way of life, and yet this again is not a true definition. For me, I realise that it is life itself. It is life in its most exciting and exacting form. It is rather as I would imagine a bird would learn how to fly, trying out its wings before hesitantly taking that first giant move into the unknown, and feeling the air gently lifting it from all that it was familiar with, but gently showing it how to be in total control of life – to soar effortlessly above time and life itself – to be totally free to reach out and take all that you desired to attain total fulfilment in every aspect – to rise above life as hitherto acknowledged, and to accept that that life existed before it became matter, before conception – to know that you, that most unique and exceptional being, was part of the universe in timelessness, long before the embryo was formed. To understand this, and to accept that your own life force was in being before conception, is a realisation of enormous magnitude that will alter your acceptance of life as you had previously known it.

This is not something that can be taught. A catalyst can explain and assist, but each person can only truly understand when they are ready to do so. I believe that when you are ready for greater awareness you will be shown the way just as birds migrate, they are not told where to go – they just know. It is like falling in love. It cannot be explained but when it happens you will know it beyond any doubt.

What can be more dramatic than the knowledge of having learned to heal ourselves through our own power. Life energy works in three ways, from consciousness to intelligence, from emotion to ecstasy and from energy to spirit. Life is ever changing. Nothing will be permanent. We must take responsibility for all that we are, and the potential for all that we wish to do is ours, and limitless until eternity. The metamorphic technique has shown me that the ultimate choice is up to life, and I am that life.

Reiki

The first time that I heard the word Reiki it conjured up a vision that was small, neat and bright, and when I learned that it was Japanese I was satisfied with my definition, as this was how I felt about these oriental people. REI means universal and KI means life energy (the natural energy within us and around us).

It has five principles:-
1. Just for today do not worry.
2. Just for today do not anger.
3. Earn your living honestly.
4. Honour your parents, teachers and elders.
5. Show gratitude to every living thing.

In the last century, Dr. Mikao Usui , a Japanese Christian Professor of Theology, searched for an explanation of how Christ and Buddha healed people by the laying on of hands. The Reiki method of natural healing is mentioned in the ancient history of Japan and the Buddhist sutras (sacred writings), and its origin goes back at least two thousand five hundred years. It was abandoned and then lost because the Zen Buddhist monks found it inadequate as the person was still (they believed) sick of spirit after the physical body had been healed. Today Reiki therapists are aware of the need to heal the individual on all levels; body, mind and soul to truly accomplish a wholistic healing. They are uncovering ancient methods and integrating them in a wholistic approach.

Reiki is neither a religion nor a belief system. The practitioner giving the treatment is just the channel for Reiki; it is the energy that does the healing. It activates, directs and applies natural energy to the promotion of healing, balance and wholeness. It assists the body's natural healing powers to relax, restore and maintain a state of well being.

When Margaret offered to give me a Reiki treatment I knew how fortunate I was to have this lovely person continue to assist me to an even higher level of good health that I had already achieved

She asked me to lie down and make myself comfortable, and she would move around me and place her hands in several pre-determined positions on my body, therefore sending energy to the whole body. On the afternoon of my initiation to Reiki I was feeling fit and happy, but confident that after my hours session I would feel even better.

To me the therapist is equally as important as the therapy and I asked Margaret to explain everything to me, and her own personal way of treating an individual. She said that although she was not taught this as part of the Reiki tradition, before commencing she said her own personal prayer that the person she was about to endeavour to help would only receive from the Highest of light and love, and that what healing was appropriate at this time would happen. I thought these simple words exactly right as I closed my eyes and expectantly faced a new beginning.

Margaret put a cloth over my eyes before covering them gently with her hands. I was immediately aware of the power in her hands, in what initially seemed to me like a variation of the Bates method of eye palming. It did have the same relaxing effect, but to a greater degree. This did not surprise me as the good of any therapy done by myself to myself was always enhanced when carried out by a caring therapist. My eyes became relaxed in the darkness, and Margaret said that she noticed a tingling in her fingers, and stayed longer on my eyes than she would normally. She then placed her hands on the top of my head for five minutes, which she said was peaceful and then on my chin, which felt as it should. On placing her hands on my throat she knew that it felt different and that there was a change in energy – she just instinctively knew that something was not quite right. She covered my ears which transported me – as always – to the joys of the seashore and childhood days of listening to the sighs of the sea in shells. It was with regret when she removed me from my daydreams, and I was instantly aware of the wind howling around the house, and the relentless drumming of the rain lashing the window panes. I was soon brought back to the reality of the moment as Margaret gently lifted my head and cradled it in her hands. She then began to massage the base of my skull firmly and gently with two fingers of each hand for an ecstatic few minutes. I had never experienced anything quite like it. The sound of the rain drifted away, and the inky blackness of my closed eyes only enhanced the energising shock waves that emanated from her fingers to spread all over my head and shoulders. It was almost sensual, and the sheer bliss of those few minutes will be a part of me forever. She then placed her hands on the top of my chest in a V shape for a full five minutes, then on to my ribs, first on one side and then the other using two hands. I must admit I was hardly aware of this as I was still on a "high" from my head massage. As Margaret placed her hands on my stomach – again in a V shape – she noticed a movement of energy, and by this time I was so relaxed and completely enveloped in the warmth and peace of a profound feeling of well-being that I was hardly aware of her words. As in a dream state I was conscious of her hands on my hips, and then on my thighs. Intuitively she placed her hands on my knees, and was not surprised when I told her that I had had arthritis in both knees many years ago. I was most impressed that she had picked up this defect, as I had cured myself so long ago that any previous pain was almost forgotten. She placed her hands on my shins and ankles before I was to turn to allow her to start on the back of my body. She started on my shoulders – two hands on one side and then on the other. Then came the thoracic area, with hands placed on either side, before moving to either side of my waist, hips, thighs, calves and ankles.

I was brought back to reality by Margaret giving a firm massage to the base of my heel, and then the ball of my foot. These were moves to bring me back to the present without altering the state of deep relaxation that I now had when I was totally free of all tension, and yet in no way giving any discordant note to the hour which had passed so fleetingly. Margaret then gently pulled on each of my toes before squeezing up the back of my leg once then giving it three upward strokes. This was to get the blood circulating, and it gave shock waves up the whole of my body so quickly that they passed out of my head like an electric current, but gave me such an alive feeling that I was vibrant. This was repeated on the other leg, causing the same feeling of life force in a way that I had never experienced before. It was exquisite! The palm of my hand was then massaged in the same firm way, and my arm squeezed three times and given three upward strokes, and then the other hand and arm was given the same treatment. Again I felt the delicious shock waves as on my legs, but not quite so electric, but decidedly exciting. Margaret then placed her hand at the top of my spine, creating a bridge with her divided fingers – the thumb and index finger together on one side of the spine, and the remaining three fingers together on the other. She then drew her hand down my spine three times from top to bottom. This gave a tingling sensation that fanned out into the whole of my back, before I had a final massage around my shoulder blades and the tops of my shoulders.

The magical hour had flown by. I had been fit and happy to start with, but now I was even more so, glowing with the pleasure received that had far outweighed any of my expectations. I had thought that after experiencing the metamorphic technique, that nothing could give me such a perfect feeling of complete calm and well being. I was wrong. In a completely different way Reiki had also done this. I have heard Reiki described as the energy which forms the basis of life. To me it is in the truest sense of the word a healing energy, leading to greater individual harmony and attunement to the basic forces of the universe. This harmony makes one whole and healthy again, and encourages the natural ability of a patient to heal himself. In Reiki treatment, use is made solely of a neutral but concentrated form of cosmic energy. With joy I realised that Reiki is a way of love, all embracing and totally good, and under Margaret's hands through which flowed her own special faith I knew that I was the most fortunate of people. With the goodness of Reiki I knew that I was cocooned in a protective shell that nothing could penetrate.

Without hesitation I had given myself into Margaret's hands completely. Confident that the inherent goodness in her would pass through her hands into my receptive self. She had the confidence of her convictions and this was important to me. I never accept only the written word but that which is proven by a person with whom I feel instant rapport. Margaret and myself both share the joy and excitement that each day brings, and the happiness that can come with sharing this love of life with others. I shall always be grateful to her for teaching me the art and science of healing and balancing the body, mind and spirit that is Reiki.

Over the years I have realised how much help I have been given from many people belonging to Dudley Cancer Support Group. It has truly been a case of the singer not the song that has been important, from our co-ordinator Diane, who is compassionate and supportive and always gives me a warm welcome, to helpers like Sue, Mary and John who have willingly given me their assistance whenever I have asked for it, and always been willing to find the answer to any of my queries. Of course we have many social events, and I have the pleasure of meeting friends regularly. Nora, who will always lend a sympathetic ear; Mary, who is quiet and serious and shares my appreciation of good reading and opera; Iris, who is full of fun, and Ethel the extrovert. All these people and many more make for happy hours spent together.

Our centre has been expanded and refurbished to become the light friendly rooms that they are today, and for me they will always be dear as all are full of echoes of Lesley.

From all diverse places I gleaned knowledge to help me relax. I recalled an interview with American tennis player Billie Jean King in the year that she helped Martina Navratilova win one of her many Wimbledon championships. I was surprised that she was not part of the group helping Martina by endeavouring to improve her tennis, but more to give her security and love, and that the one thing that she must never forget was the tennis ball. Everything hinged on it to the point that Billie Jean put tennis balls at random all around Martina's home, so that she was constantly reminded of its importance. The idea was that when she was on court and under extreme pressure she would think of those times at home, in tranquillity where a tennis ball seemed to be everywhere. The important point was that she and Billie Jean made a fun thing of it, and this would subliminally now affect her game when it was most needed. I was impressed with Billie Jean's psychology, and a happy and relaxed Martina when interviewed after winning her title confirmed what Billie Jean had said. I was sure that this constant putting the right thoughts into the mind in a loved environment was an inimitable idea from which I would find my own parallel. At various places around the house I put myself little messages to relax, as this was what I most needed to learn to accomplish, and I had to admit over the ensuing weeks that they did help. My natural instincts were to become tense under pressure, and the unobtrusive note that I would glimpse would remind me not to as I passed from one part of the house to another. Billie Jean was right when she said that constant reminders were needed of something important to be learned and totally mastered, and I decided that if Martina could do it in front of a Wimbledon crowd and thousands of television viewers, then I could surely emulate her in the quiet of my home. It is still hard to do, but I give it my best efforts, and I know that I am winning. Every situation that in the past would cause instant tension but in which I can now help myself to stay calm is a plus point for me, and helps me to attain even more successes, until I reach the ultimate goal of being able to control my heart rhythm automatically.

For many years I had appreciated the value of Doctor Bach's Rescue Remedy, and thought I would ask for more specific advice, as I wanted to do all that I could to help my body heal itself. I contacted the principal consultant Judy Howard of the Doctor E. Bach Centre, who listened while I explained that my heart condition had prompted me to contact her, although I appreciated that the Bach remedies were for the whole person, which I believed implicitly was the only way to rectify any bodily imperfections. After asking questions about me she suggested that I try three remedies – Aspen for apprehension, as I so easily became tense for no real reason, Vervain for being an admitted workaholic – so easy to be one when there are not enough hours in the day to do all that I wanted to – and also to help my highly strung nature, causing tension, and Olive for my feelings of being drained of energy and for finding some days just too much to cope with, leaving me fatigued. I was to take two drops of each in spring water at least four times a day and sipping it slowly as and when I felt it necessary. I had no intention of becoming dependent on anything, but I had such high regard for Doctor Bach's philosophy and the worth of his Rescue Remedy that I was certain that this specific prescription for me would aid me through any difficult days and besides – just knowing that it was in my small medicine bag gave me a sense of security.

I now have a wealth of knowledge to assist me in my ever

widening vision of gaining perfect health. Always I will live by the maxim that any illness that can be prevented I will prevent. What ailments I succumb to I will cure if they are curable – and only by the most natural means available. If by some misfortune I ever have something that I cannot vanquish – and not only by orthodox diagnosis but by my own acceptance of fact – then I will ensure that all that it is possible to do to assist my condition will be done, in all the natural palliative methods that I know. Knowing that most bodily imbalances can be eradicated, and everything can be helped, the future holds no fears. No ailment shall be treated as an isolated part of me, but as a manifestation of a whole that is showing external symptoms that need attention and help to the whole body. To me the familiar adjectives of alternative and complimentary do not fit into my new life-style. I use the word "natural" as all the healing help that I use and the daily routine that I have worked out for myself are all that is wholesome, full of goodness and entirely natural. All of this I know to be true, and the allure of radiant health will always take me forward along the path of fitness. Every day I shall be glad to be alive, glad to be healthy, glad to be a person who is aware of all life's precious gifts. I will cling to my way of life and make every moment bright with health and happiness. My attention was drawn to the words of Henrik Ibsen "Think, work, act, don't sit here and brood amongst insoluble enigmas" and this is sound advice. Always remember – *This is the day which the Lord hath made; we will rejoice and be glad in it. PS 118:24.*

21

GRIEF

Ideally a New Year should be heralded with all trumpets sounding and great happiness and achievement to be enjoyed. Nineteen ninety one arrived with gale's of unimaginable ferocity the amalgam of which caused havoc throughout our country. So much of the world is in hostilities against other nations and I see the futility of young healthy lives over before they have a chance to live. In my own world so many of my friends have lost their fight for life after unceasing struggle.

My dear friend Lesley died of liver cancer in a bleak cold January when the dampness of the air and the moisture from the trees that she so loved shed tears for her. She had been unwell towards the end of nineteen ninety and had been forced to discontinue our regular meetings. In December she telephoned to suggest that we meet at the Group's Christmas party and it was with much eagerness that I agreed. As always the room was light and cheerful and on this night brightly decorated and filled with laughter and chatter with a traditional seasonal buffet for our added enjoyment. Over the years I had learned to mask my feelings and this served me well as Lesley came towards me. The thick vibrant hair was now dull and lank and the rounded cheeks hollowed and drawn. Her eyes were sunken, and lack lustre where they had once glowed warm and brown. She was a travesty of the girl that I had last seen and only the sonorous voice was the same as she hugged me, as I realised that this time there was no escape for her. The day of her funeral was a day of unnatural stillness as if all nature was in silence out of respect for her passing. The earth was rock hard and my park pond, refrozen nightly after never quite thawing in those cold days, gave a miniature scene of barren arctic frozen waste of icy pulchritude relieved only by small patches of crystallised snow still remaining from flurries of many days ago, and the strange footprints of small birds etched on the coldness. The scene was no bleaker than the emptiness that I felt at having to accept that the earthly life of Lesley was finally over.

At times life is an enigma to me in that such treasured people who have so much to give to others should die, and when young men go proudly to war that I do not see as glory but pointless destruction of a most precious life. I continue, learning all the time and in some ways untouched by any evil and unbitter for what I have lost; just grateful for the privilege of having shared precious moments with such personages who continue to enrich my life even when their own brightly flickering candle has been extinguished forever. I do not question these sad events. If you give all that you can during your friends' lifetime you need have no regret at their passing and sadness at their loss becomes a happy memory bathed in a serene aura of sunshine – just as their lives were when they touched mine. I am always seeking and learning, welcoming sharing my life with good people.

Learning to accept the loss of dear ones is one of life's hardest lessons to learn. When I was young I would say to my mother that I wanted to die when she did, but as she wisely said, we had not come together and it was doubtful that we would go together, and that we came into the world alone and we would die alone. Initially it is sometimes difficult not to feel bitterness and resentment that such an unacceptable loss has to happen as to lose the person that meant the whole world to you, and life is unendurable without that person. The overwhelming assailance of grief that follows is nature's way of healing. Shared grief can bring comfort, and to cry in the secure love of family or close friends is the way to gain the strength to continue with life. Never go against nature's wishes and keep emotions pent up inside an already tortured body. Cry alone if this is the chosen way, and only time will help. It is said that God takes the best people for his own and it so often seems like that as the dearest of people are those that are taken away from us. Find some solace in that they are out of all pain and are at peace, and are looking at us from their new and perfect lives, and they do not wish us to remain sad forever. It is not always easy to understand the ways of God, but we must not question that He knows best, and over the months and the years you will find with shock that you can laugh and be happy and look forward to a life without that beloved person. The memory that remains grows ever warmer and never dims at all.With the passing of the emotional floods the peace will come, and you will be glad you shared in the life of the dear one, and feel no bitterness that you are no longer together on this earth, because you will always be together in spirit. This is one of the hardest crosses of all to bear but they are all part of the life that God has given us and with fortitude He makes us strong enough to carry the burdens He puts in our paths. Just reflect, and you will realise that the people who have lost the most and suffered greatly are those who seem the most happy and contented and full of joy and generous in love for everyone.

To have loved a person who dies of a terminal illness years before his time is sad, but nothing is like the shock of having a fit person die in tragic circumstances. A year ago Gwen, a dear lady who had been like a kindly aunt all of my life was killed in a car accident. A treasured life was blotted out in seconds, leaving a loving family numbed by shock. Val, a friend of mine for over a quarter of a century, was also killed in a horrific car accident. She of the soft voice and sweet caring nature of whom I never heard utter a harsh word of anyone, even when life treated her unkindly, was another life over. The shock waves engulfing those of us left who loved them will be with us for a lifetime. Val's brother Barrie said that the world will be a poorer place without his sister and these wise words are true, and even though we know that these people are at peace, we are left with empty places where they should be, and it is hard to accept. All the memories of such people are good, kind and caring and full of happiness. Such are these precious people.

First grief comes for most of us as children – and it certainly did for me – when a beloved pet dies. A pet who has been a companion and friend and playmate during ones early years – the sadness of burying a lifeless body in a garden where once you played together – a little grave tended faithfully. As the years go on the pain lessens into a distant childhood memory but to me losing my cat Blackie was the first stage of growing up, and my first sad moment in a happy childhood. My father's wartime hens were also playmates of my early years, accepting me into their pen where I played in the dust as they scratched contentedly. They did not appear to mind as I chased them around the lawn, shreaking noisily. Daily they came to greet me and suffered my small fingers to ruffle their soft feathers. As each one died I was sad at their loss, until over the years they were all gone.

We must not let grief take over our lives but bask in the happy memories that nothing can erase, and in the sure knowledge that one day we shall be reunited with all the beloved people and pets who have gone before us.

The following poem gives comfort with its simple words:-

Do not stand at my grave and weep
I am not there. I do not sleep.
I am a thousand winds that blow
I am the diamond glints on snow.
I am the sunlight on ripened grain
I am the gentle autumn rain.
When you awaken in the morning 's hush
I am the swift uplifting rush
of quiet birds in circled flight.
I am the soft stars that shine at night.
Do not stand at my grave and cry,
I am not there; I did not die.

22

SELF LOVE

Many people over the years who have taken note of my full life have commented that I rarely if ever give any time to myself. So busy am I being a daughter, wife, mother and friend that thinking of myself in a caring way has just never entered my mind as being of necessity. I realise looking over my shoulder at all the hard years of learning and piecing my life's picture, that I have missed out a most important piece – loving myself. It is realising suddenly that I have collected all the ingredients of the best quality, but missed out one vital component to complete the recipe. So often I am asked why I don't make a life for myself. This did not mean the time spent on becoming well again or rushing about on empty pleasures, but pausing and thinking about myself.

I had worked so hard that deep down I must have felt I was worth it. I must learn to pamper myself. If my body enjoyed and flourished when given the most nourishing foods, then my whole being must be given love, consideration, affection and happiness for me to be truly complete. I was in no way dissatisfied and was aware of all the good things in my life, but I never felt of myself in a loving way. Love to me was to be given to others, never to myself. This was so unique that it did take a long time before I considered myself automatically prior to accepting an impossibly restricting schedule that left me too tired to give even a thought to my willing and obliging body, that had helped me over the years. It was my turn now to return that devotion, until I was merged into a totally loving being. Caring for myself did not mean in any way to be selfish, just to make myself a more complete person, who in turn would be more loving to others. The smile that I gave to others made me feel good, the shared laughter even better.

I began to start the day aware that I was full of all powerful, forceful radiating love that flowed constantly, and all the personal care now given to myself took on a new dimension. Washing was done with care to make my body as clean as possible; dressing was done to make my body as warm and comfortable as required, so that it would be contented. My hair would be daily brushed in firm rhythmic strokes, and the bristles would caress my scalp and make it strong from which would grow glossy hair. My mind was never subjected to harsh noise – only music that fed the soul deep within me and my eyes would never be subjected to over bright light – only the gentle-health giving daylight and radiance of sunlight that was pure, and entered my being with its benevolent rays. My home is uncluttered with garish items that would jar and grate on my person – only special treasures – objects made by Jamie when small and so carefully brought from early school days and given to me with such love – little gifts treasured when their reminder brings joy that they were given to me from dear people. I find time to be myself – to give myself space – sometimes just to sit in the summer sunshine, or sometimes to do what I want to do – write a letter to a friend whom I rarely see and have so much love to send, or create a special place in my garden because I shall derive so much pleasure in seeing it flourish and mature into an area born of communication with the earth.

I make plans that will make me happy, for it is always good to have something to look forward to, but I live only in the present. I let the past go and bear no resentment for past hurts. I remember only the good and the warmth of past friendships still enters my receptive body and I am content. Have no fears for the future. It is unlikely that it will come as you think it may. Love every day and make time to love yourself. Always hang on to your dreams and most of them will come true – not perhaps in the way that you thought they would, but perfectly unfolding in a different way, and full of love as you recognise and hold out your arms to embrace the future that is there for you to curl your gentle fingers round. All that you wish for will come to you, for nothing is more worthy of the best in life than a person full of love. Always take time to love yourself for all love is a God given privilege and quintessential. Loving yourself genuinely gives a quiet tranquillity of peace and perfect balance, and the erstwhile age of childhood contentment will be yours again. Love is at the heart of life and your love for yourself is at the heart of your life and fills it until you are enveloped in happiness. Remember the words of Bertrand Russell *"Love is everything. All the rest is standing on the edge and staring into the abyss"*.

In the late nineteen sixties an American psychologist named Aaron Beck introduced cognitive therapy, the aim of which was to boost self-confidence, by learning to believe in yourself. It could be practised alone or in groups, but it always sought to discard all negative and unworthy thoughts and in their place put positive feelings, which would assist in having a high regard for oneself. When mastered, self worth would prevail, and this would inevitably be followed by a joy of living in which all things were good. Any such feeling radiated to encompass all with whom such a person came into contact, and love and satisfaction with oneself was achieved. I found it most gratifying to have learned that self-love was considered sufficiently necessary to be actually a therapy, and to me it would always be of paramount importance.

The French have an old saying that explains how your life is divided into three parts. The first is for growing; the second is for working and the third is for living. I make sure now that my life is for living, with unstinting love for myself and for everyone. This is the secret of true health, happiness and contentment.

Many soubriquets can be attached to my lifestyle but there is no enigma, just living a life of probity and never letting good be subjugated by tainted reason. A penchant for striving to learn all of life that I can and turning everything to an advantage is always dominated by love – nothing profane – only love.

These words are no idle soliloquy nor the musing of a somnambulist, but the realisation that I must accept my own worth unfettered by any trivia. It is almost like accepting a mantra of life, and the need of its power that would be eternal as the sweeps of a windmill endlessly turning in rhythmic beats. This is no brief illusion but the knowledge that I had recognised and understood something so precious that it would always be mine.

*Let the star of the morning shine on you every day of
your life.
Trust in its brightness and love and protection for it is
always there if you will only look upwards and see it.*

I look back over the years of heartache and struggle since
those long-ago days when I first learned to become aware of
life's evolution, and how after many mistakes and false starts I
had become the person that I now was – better in health than
I had been for years and full of optimism for the future. No
day passed that I did not pray to God in gratitude for showing
me the path on which to go, and guiding me with heightened
instincts in the proper direction. I have so much to live for
and so much to be thankful for that I go forward with assur-
ance, knowing that I will always treasure the great gift of life.
Only time will tell if I have made the right choices, but in my
heart I know that I have, and I shall know the answer with
patience, because truth is the daughter of time.

EPILOGUE

It seems exactly right that my final words should be of the Bristol Cancer Help Centre as it was that pioneering book *The Bristol Diet* by Dr. Alec Forbes that was the first step in teaching me how to help myself get well again. On a bright day in early spring when my park was covered in a dusty haze of the palest mauve crocuses, and the sun shone on the opaque white flowers of the hawthorn giving it a pale golden glow as the sun lightly touched the lemon stamens, I was glad to be alive with the chills of winter past and a promised hot summer before me.

With eager anticipation I had arranged to meet Liz, representative of the Bristol Cancer Help Centre, who was spending a day with our Group. Liz was a fit looking person as I would have expected, and keen to know how she could help me. I produced my well thumbed copy of *The Bristol Diet* and briefly explained how it had been the initiation to the good health that I now enjoyed. As I had expected she was interested to hear of the years of help I had derived from it – which she informed me was out of print and now a collectors item. I assured her that I would never part with it. Why should I? I owed my life to its wise words.

I said that what I really wanted was an updating of the diet recommended by the Centre. When I explained my own regime that was so satisfactory and enjoyable to me she could only commend my perseverance in establishing such a suitable diet for myself with which I was happy to live. Her advice was to continue just the way that I was. She remarked on how well I looked; this was music to my ears, and I was more than pleased when she informed me that she would be forwarding any updated information to Diane, who could pass it on to me. She also suggested that I might find Rose Elliot's book *The Green Age Diet* interesting, and I promised to secure myself a copy of this unheard of volume. She thought my willingness to eat healthily and keep in tune to the dictates of my body, plus my open-mindedness to anything newly discovered could not be improved upon. She asked whether I ate organically and I said I did at every opportunity, particularly carrots which I was able to obtain. It was obvious that she had far more outlets in Bristol than I had here in Dudley for healthy produce. We both agreed that bean sprouts were excellent but she understood when I said they did not figure in my diet as often as I would wish due to the time-consuming nature of their preparation. She volunteered that people often lost weight on this type of diet, and was interested when I said that I had actually put on over a stone, which is exactly what I had aimed to do. I asked her whether she ate healthily or took supplements and of course she did eat as well as she was able and only took a multivitamin tablet a day which she had found beneficial, particularly after illness. She told me that the Centre recommended vitamin C supplements to its patients, as it was impossible to overdose, as the body was able to rid itself of any surplus of this vitamin. I told her that I felt my diet adequately provided for all the vitamins including vitamin C, and she accepted that my diet was good. She admitted to a weakness for chocolate, and I told her that I doubted that she could be more addicted than I used to be, but could truthfully say that I did not crave it any longer.

In meeting a representative of the Bristol Cancer Help Centre at this point in my life when I felt that I had found all the pieces of my life's jigsaw and by my own endeavours, and the help of many people, I could now fit everything in harmoniously. I felt the wheel had come full circle in ending as it started with *The Bristol Diet* book. In the last seven years I can hardly believe that I have come so far and learned so much, and found such pleasure in a great deal of it. This is no erudite work, but my own personal story, written mainly for my friends of Dudley Cancer Support Group, who have given me their unique help, in an endeavour to help any of them who wish to assist by their own efforts to recapture that elusive commodity – their own good health.

Over the years so many people have exclaimed at how from being so unwell I have regained my fitness, and everyday I become stronger and can look forward to a life unshackled by any bodily imbalance. Many years have now passed and all the time my energy is renewed and the future holds all that is good. I have no time to be unwell. This is how I achieved Good Health.